THE

CARBOHYDRATE

ADDICT'S GRAM

COUNTER

DR. RICHARD F. HELLER
PROFESSOR, MT. SINAI SCHOOL OF MEDICINE • PROFESSOR, GRADUATE CENTER OF THE CITY UNIVERSITY OF NEW YORK • PROFESSOR EMERITUS, CITY UNIVERSITY OF NEW YORK

DR. RACHAEL F. HELLER
ASSISTANT PROFESSOR, MT. SINAI SCHOOL OF MEDICINE • ASSISTANT CLINICAL PROFESSOR, GRADUATE CENTER OF THE CITY UNIVERSITY OF NEW YORK

⊘
A SIGNET BOOK

SIGNET

Published by New American Library, a division of
Penguin Putnam Inc., 375 Hudson Street,
New York, New York 10014, U.S.A.
Penguin Books Ltd, 27 Wrights Lane, London W8 5TZ, England
Penguin Books Australia Ltd, Ringwood, Victoria, Australia
Penguin Books Canada Ltd, 10 Alcorn Avenue, Toronto, Ontario, Canada M4V 3B2
Penguin Books (N.Z.) Ltd, 182–190 Wairau Road, Auckland 10, New Zealand

Penguin Books Ltd, Registered Offices: Harmondsworth, Middlesex, England

First published by Signet, an imprint of New American Library,
a division of Penguin Putnam Inc.

First Printing, June 1993
19

CONTENTS

*Nutritional values in this counter were taken from material supplied by or direct communication with the U.S. Department of Agriculture, The U.S. Center for Disease Control, scientific journal articles, computer data banks, and representatives of the food industry.

CONTENTS

INTRODUCTION

Are You A Carbohydrate Addict?

Do you love breads and other starches, snack foods or sweets? Do you find you can't stop eating them once you start? Do you eat too much of them—in spite of what you have promised yourself? If so, chances are you are a carbohydrate addict. Something in your body responds differently to that bread or pasta or potato, to those snack foods or sweets, than it does to celery or lettuce or to cauliflower.

Let's face it, when we bite into an eclair or a warm piece of bread our body feels good—very good—and no green bean brings about the same response.

Science is finally recognizing that when it comes to eating and weight, as in many other physical processes, everyone is *not* the same. C. Everett Koop, M.D., the former Surgeon General of the United States calls us "carbohydrate sensitive." Researchers have shown that up to 75% of the overweight (and many normal-weight individuals as well) are carbohydrate addicts. Thousands of scientists have documented the metabolic imbalance that causes us to have carbohydrate cravings and makes us more likely to put on weight, to keep it on, and to regain it if it is lost through dieting. The bad news is that we are carbohydrate addicts; our genes have made us carbohydrate sensitive and no matter how great our willpower, at times our bodies fight us every step of the way. The good news is that we now know what causes carbohydrate addiction and, best of all, how to correct it.

<u>Carbohydrate addiction is *not* a matter of willpower;</u>
<u>it is a matter of biology.</u>

If you are a carbohydrate addict you may find that:

> You have difficulty stopping once you've started to eat bread, pasta or other starches, snack foods or sweets

> After you've had a full breakfast, you get hungrier before it's time for lunch than if you had skipped breakfast or had only a cup of coffee

You get tired and/or hungry in the midafternoon

You have a tendency to put on weight easily, to keep it on, and to regain it if it is lost through dieting

You lose control of your eating; regularly or on occasion

Bread or other starches, snack foods or sweets have been your diet downfall

If you are a carbohydrate addict, we understand why you have struggled to stay on diets and why diet after diet has failed to keep the weight off. Carbohydrate-rich foods hold the key to addiction for the carbohydrate-sensitive person. While on our program these foods can be enjoyed every day, in satisfying and pleasurable quantities, but the guidelines for doing so must be understood. For basic diet guidelines for carbohydrate addicts, see our first book, *The Carbohydrate Addict's Diet* (Signet).

WHAT THIS BOOK WILL DO FOR YOU

Calories, Carbohydrates and Fats: In the sections that follow, you will find the calorie, carbohydrate, and fat contents for 2,700 foods. We have included a wide variety of foods—those we eat every day and those that may be a bit more unusual. They are easy to locate and to read.

Healthy Heart (♥)
Calories, carbohydrates, and fats do not always tell you what is actually in your food or how it will affect you. Manufacturers are allowed to report caloric, carbohydrate, and fat levels with room for errors of up to 20% from the actual content. For these reasons, we have included a Healthy Heart symbol (♥) to help you easily locate foods that are lower in fat levels.

In order to receive our Healthy Heart symbol, foods must contain no more than 20% of calories in fat (as per many current health recommendations) and, in addition, foods must not be so high in calories that high levels of fat may be hidden within them. We have not awarded our Healthy Heart to that class of questionable foods (including alcohol and food-replacement drinks) which, while they do not contain high levels of fat, do not necessarily qualify for a "healthy heart."

Trigger Foods (T)

Although carbohydrate addicts can, within our guidelines, eat all foods and remain free of carbohydrate cravings and weight concerns, Trigger Foods should be confined to Reward Meals (see *The Carbohydrate Addict's Diet*). Trigger Foods are foods which are usually not recognized as being high in carbohydrates, but which have repeatedly been shown to bring on carbohydrate cravings, hunger, and weight gain and we have awarded them their own special symbol (T). Some Trigger Foods are high in carbohydrates but they fool dieters. Often, these foods are perceived as "healthy" or "diet" foods and dieters do not pay attention to their high carbohydrate levels. Foods such as fruits and juices, yogurt, pita bread, even carrots and broccoli, fall into this group. Other Trigger Foods such as medications or additives are low in carbohydrates but seem to cause metabolic changes in the body that result in cravings or weight gain (or both). Included in this group are alcohol, artificial sweeteners, and monosodium glutamate. In the listings that follow, be on the lookout for our trigger symbol: T; some Trigger Foods are sure to surprise you.

Easy Comparison

We have made comparison between foods and between brands simple. Whenever possible, we have standardized portions so that you will be comparing, for instance, 3 ounces of beef to 3 ounces of chicken. You can now easily identify your choices in terms of calories, carbohydrates, or fat. The information that you need is there—at a glance.

In general, when many different companies package the same foods or when several different recipes are used, we have averaged the food values. When one or two companies stand out as having high or low values on the same foods, we have included them by name so that you are free to make your choice. Food values have been rounded off to the nearest tenth or whole number.

REAL-LIFE CHOICES— SPECIAL SECTIONS
DESIGNED TO MEET *YOUR* NEEDS

Eating Out—Ethnic Style

What you need to know about your favorite ethnic food: Chinese, Italian, Deli, Mexican, Japanese, French, and Middle-Eastern. Food values are given on sandwiches, whole platters and dinners, along with separate food items.

Fast Food Restaurants

Want to compare a Whopper with a Big Mac? It's easy, just look it up. A full array of the most popular fast-food fare is at your fingertips.

Salad Bar and Dressings

A complete listing of salad bar fixings and dressings.

Medications

Did you know that as many as five different sugars can be found in one vitamin tablet? Did you know that some pain relievers or cough syrups can cause carbohydrate cravings and weight gain? This important section will arm you with essential information.

Vegetarian Choices, Meat, Dairy, Fish and Poultry Substitutes

A full array of non-meat and low-fat options provide delicious alternatives to meat, dairy, fish, and poultry.

A SPECIAL NOTE TO OUR READERS

Any change in diet should be made in consultation with your physician. Trigger and Healthy Heart symbols are given as informational data only. They are not intended to replace medical advice. Any questions or concerns should be addressed to your physician.

We hope that this counter will become a good and well-used friend. It carries with it the experiences of over a quarter of a million people along with our best wishes for a long and healthy life.

Item	SERVING	CAL-ORIES	CARBS (g)	TOTAL FAT(g)	♥	T
Amaretto	1 fl. oz.	76	9	0.0		T
Apple juice	8 fl. oz.	115	29	0.0	♥	T
Apricot cordial	1 fl. oz.	79	8	0.0		T
Apricot nectar	8 fl. oz.	140	36	0.0	♥	T
Beer						
light	8 fl. oz.	63	3	0.0		T
regular	8 fl. oz.	167	7	0.0		T
Breakfast drink, instant*						
chocolate						
no sugar	1 env.	70	10	1.0	♥	T
regular	1 env.	130	25	1.0	♥	
chocolate malt						
no sugar	1 env.	70	8	2.0		T
regular	1 env.	130	24	2.0	♥	
strawberry						
no sugar	1 env.	70	10	0.3	♥	T
regular	1 env.	130	25	0.2	♥	
vanilla						
no sugar	1 env.	70	10	0.2	♥	T
regular	1 env.	130	25	0.2	♥	
Carrot juice	8 fl. oz.	97	23	0.4	♥	T
Champagne	3½ fl. oz.	87	0	0.0		T
Clam & tomato cocktail	8 fl. oz.	107	25	0.0	♥	
Club soda	8 fl. oz.	0	0	0.0	♥	
Cocoa						
w/low-fat milk powder	8 fl. oz.	133	29	1.3	♥	
w/whole milk	8 fl. oz.	225	30	9.0		
Coffee	8 fl. oz.	0	0	0.0	♥	
Coffees, flavored						
(Gen. Foods International)						
Cafe Amaretto	8 fl. oz.	67	9	2.7		
Cafe Francais						
regular	8 fl. oz.	80	8	4.0		
sugar-free	8 fl. oz.	47	4	2.7		T
Cafe Irish Creme	8 fl. oz.	67	11	2.7		
Cafe Vienna						
regular	8 fl. oz.	80	13	2.7		
sugar-free	8 fl. oz.	40	4	2.7		T
Chocolate Double-Dutch	8 fl. oz.	67	11	2.7		
Chocolate Mint Dutch	8 fl. oz.	67	11	2.7		

♥ = HEALTHY HEART FOOD T = TRIGGER FOOD
*Only values for dry ingredient are given; add calories, carbohydrates, and fat for added regular or lower fat milk.

Item	SERVING	CAL-ORIES	CARBS (g)	TOTAL FAT(g)	♥	T
Orange Cappuccino						
regular	8 fl. oz.	80	13	2.7		
sugar-free	8 fl. oz.	40	4	2.7		T
Suisse Mocha						
regular	8 fl. oz.	67	9	4.0		
sugar-free	8 fl. oz.	40	4	2.7		T
Coffee-flavor grain bev.	8 fl. oz.	13	3	0.0	♥	
Coke						
regular	8 fl. oz.	101	27	0.0	♥	
sugar-free (Diet Coke)	8 fl. oz.	1	0	0.0	♥	T
Cola						
regular	8 fl. oz.	107	27	0.0	♥	
sugar-free	8 fl. oz.	0	0	0.0	♥	T
Cranberry juice cocktail	8 fl. oz.	147	35	0.0	♥	
Cranberry juice, sweetened	8 fl. oz.	145	38	0.0	♥	
Creme de Cacao	1 fl. oz.	96	13	0.0		T
Creme de Menthe	1 fl. oz.	96	12	0.0		T
Crystal Light						
iced tea	8 fl. oz.	2	0	0.0	♥	T
most flavors	8 fl. oz.	2	0	0.0	♥	T
Dr Pepper						
diet	8 fl. oz.	2	0	0.0	♥	T
regular	8 fl. oz.	107	27	0.0	♥	
Eggnog	8 fl. oz.	340	30	19.0		
Fruit punch drink	8 fl. oz.	113	30	0.0	♥	
Gin	1½ fl. oz.	105	0	0.0		
Ginger ale						
raspberry	8 fl. oz.	87	21	0.0	♥	
raspberry, diet	8 fl. oz.	3	1	0.0	♥	T
regular	8 fl. oz.	83	21	0.0	♥	
regular, sugar-free	8 fl. oz.	3	1	0.0	♥	T
Grape drink	8 fl. oz.	133	35	0.0	♥	
Grape juice	8 fl. oz.	120	36	0.0	♥	
Grape soda	8 fl. oz.	120	31	0.0	♥	
Grapefruit juice	8 fl. oz.	96	23	0.0	♥	T
Lemonade, from concentrate	8 fl. oz.	99	27	0.0	♥	
Lemon-lime soda	8 fl. oz.	103	26	0.0	♥	
Limeade	8 fl. oz.	100	27	0.0	♥	
Liquid fasts (food replacement drinks)						
DynaTrim	8 fl. oz.	220	31	3.0		T
Ultra Slim Fast, French vanilla	11 fl. oz.	210	38	3.0		T
Ultra Slim Fast Plus w/juice	12 fl. oz.	250	57	1.0		T

♥ = HEALTHY HEART FOOD   T = TRIGGER FOOD

Item	SERVING	CAL-ORIES	CARBS (g)	TOTAL FAT(g)	♥	T
Milk						
chocolate, low fat	8 fl. oz.	170	26	4.0		
chocolate, regular	8 fl. oz.	210	26	8.0		
low fat (1%)	8 fl. oz.	100	12	3.0		T
low fat (2%)	8 fl. oz.	120	12	5.0		T
nonfat	8 fl. oz.	85	12	0.0	♥	T
skim	8 fl. oz.	85	12	0.0	♥	T
whole	8 fl. oz.	150	11	8.0		
Orange-Grapefruit juice	8 fl. oz.	105	25	0.0	♥	
Orange juice	8 fl. oz.	110	26	0.0	♥	T
Orange soda	8 fl. oz.	120	31	0.0	♥	
Pepsi						
regular	8 fl. oz.	107	26	0.0	♥	
sugar-free (Pepsi Light)	8 fl. oz.	1	0	0.0	♥	T
Pineapple-grapefruit juice	8 fl. oz.	120	31	0.0	♥	
Pineapple juice, unsweetened	8 fl. oz.	140	34	0.0	♥	
Quinine water						
regular	8 fl. oz.	75	19	0.0	♥	
sugar-free	8 fl. oz.	3	0	0.0	♥	T
Root beer						
regular	8 fl. oz.	103	27	0.0	♥	
sugar-free	8 fl. oz.	1	0	0.0	♥	T
Rum	1½ fl. oz.	105	0	0.0		
7Up						
regular	8 fl. oz.	96	24	0.0	♥	
sugar-free	8 fl. oz.	3	0	0.0	♥	T
Shake						
chocolate	8 fl. oz.	268	48	6.4		
vanilla	8 fl. oz.	252	40	7.2		
Sprite						
regular	8 fl. oz.	90	24	0.0	♥	
sugar-free	8 fl. oz.	3	0	0.0	♥	T
Tab	8 fl. oz.	1	1	0.0	♥	T
Tea						
brewed	8 fl. oz.	0	0	0.0	♥	
instant, artificially-sweetened	8 fl. oz.	1	1	0.0	♥	T
instant, sweetened	8 fl. oz.	85	22	0.0	♥	
instant, unsweetened	8 fl. oz.	0	0	0.0	♥	
Tomato juice	8 fl. oz.	40	10	0.0	♥	
Tonic water						
regular	8 fl. oz.	85	22	0.0	♥	
sugar-free	8 fl. oz.	1	0	0.0	♥	T
Yoo-Hoo, chocolate drink	8 fl. oz.	124	24	1.0	♥	

♥ = HEALTHY HEART FOOD   T = TRIGGER FOOD

Item	SERVING	CAL-ORIES	CARBS (g)	TOTAL FAT(g)	♥	T
Vegetable juice cocktail	8 fl. oz.	45	11	0.0	♥	T
Vegetable juice, V-8	8 fl. oz.	47	11	0.0	♥	T
Vodka	1½ fl. oz.	105	0	0.0		T
Whisky	1½ fl. oz.	105	0	0.0		T
Wine						
champagne	3½ fl. oz.	87	0	0.0		T
cream sherry	3½ fl. oz.	140	11	0.0		T
dessert wine	3½ fl. oz.	140	8	0.0		T
port	3½ fl. oz.	165	11	0.0		T
red wine	3½ fl. oz.	75	3	0.0		T
sherry	3½ fl. oz.	133	11	0.0		T
white wine	3½ fl. oz.	80	3	0.0		T

BREADS, CRACKERS, AND FLOURS

Item	SERVING	CAL-ORIES	CARBS (g)	TOTAL FAT(g)	♥	T
Bagels						
cinnamon & raisin	1	300	55	2.0	♥	T
egg	1	250	54	3.0	♥	
garlic/onion	1	220	43	2.0	♥	
plain	1	200	38	2.0	♥	T
poppy seed	1	205	38	2.0	♥	
Biscuits						
baking powder						
commercial	1 oz.	88	10	3.4		
homemade	1 oz.	105	13	4.9		
buttermilk						
commercial	1 oz.	115	17	3.8		
commercial, extra rich	1 oz.	130	18	6.0		
homemade	1 oz.	120	19	4.0		
plain						
from mix	1	95	14	3.0		
from refrigerator dough	1	65	10	2.0		
homemade	1	100	13	5.0		
Bread cubes	1 cup	80	15	1.0	♥	
Bread crumbs						
commercial	1 cup	390	73	5.0		
homemade	1 cup	120	22	2.0		
Breads						
brown, Boston	1 slice	95	21	1.0	♥	

♥ = HEALTHY HEART FOOD   T = TRIGGER FOOD

Item	SERVING	CAL-ORIES	CARBS (g)	TOTAL FAT(g)	♥	T
cinnamon raisin	1 slice	85	12	1.0	♥	T
cracked wheat						
commercial	1 slice	75	14	1.0	♥	
homemade	1 slice	65	12	1.0	♥	
French						
Pepperidge Farm (thick slice)	1	150	27	3.0	♥	
restaurant (thick slice)	1	101	20	1.0	♥	
Wonder	1 slice	75	14	1.0	♥	
granola, oat, & honey	1 slice	60	12	2.0	♥	T
honey bran	1 slice	90	18	1.0	♥	
Italian	1 slice	85	17	0.0	♥	
mixed grain	1 slice	65	12	1.0	♥	T
oatmeal bread	1 slice	65	12	1.0	♥	
pita bread	1 pita	165	33	1.0	♥	T
pumpernickel	1 slice	80	16	1.0	♥	
raisin	1 slice	65	13	1.0	♥	T
raisin nut	1 slice	95	15	3.0		
rye	1 slice	65	12	1.0	♥	
seven grain	1 slice	90	18	2.0		T
sour dough	1 slice	70	14	1.0	♥	
Vienna	1 slice	70	13	1.0	♥	
wheat						
commercial	1 slice	65	12	1.0	♥	
Pepperidge Farm	1 slice	95	18	1.5	♥	
white						
light	1 slice	42	10	0.5	♥	
regular	1 slice	65	12	1.0	♥	
thin	1 slice	54	10	1.0	♥	
whole wheat	1 slice	70	13	1.0	♥	
whole wheat—honey prune	1 slice	75	16	0.5	♥	T
Cornbread						
commercial	1 square	140	21	5.0		
from mix	1 square	140	21	5.0		
homemade	1 square	115	17	4.1		
Southern style	1 square	160	23	5.6		
Crackers (by the piece)						
butter thins	1 cracker	18	3	1.0		
cheese, plain	1 cracker	5	1	0.3		
cheese, sandwich	1 sandwich	40	5	2.0		
graham	1 cracker	30	6	0.5	♥	
Melba toast	1 piece	20	4	0.0	♥	
rye wafers	1 wafer	28	5	0.5	♥	
saltines	1 cracker	12	2	0.2	♥	

♥ = HEALTHY HEART FOOD   T = TRIGGER FOOD

Item	SERVING	CAL-ORIES	CARBS (g)	TOTAL FAT(g)	♥	T
wheat, thin	1 cracker	9	1	0.2		
whole wheat wafers	1 cracker	18	2	1.0		
Crackers (by weight)						
butter						
Town House	1 oz.	140	16	8.0		T
Ritz	1 oz.	140	18	8.0		T
cheese						
Cheese Nips	1 oz.	140	18	6.0		T
Goldfish	1 oz.	120	19	4.0		T
Goldfish, pizza	1 oz.	130	19	5.0		T
Ritz Bits Cheese	1 oz.	140	16	8.0		T
Oysterettes	1 oz.	120	20	2.0	♥	
peanut butter & cheese	1 oz.	136	16	6.4		T
Rykrisp	1 oz.	80	22	0.0	♥	
Rykrisp, sesame	1 oz.	100	20	2.0	♥	
saltine	1 oz.	120	20	4.0		
Sociables	1 oz.	140	18	3.0		
soda	1 oz.	140	22	4.0		
seven grain	1 oz.	110	18	4.0		T
Stoned Wheat Thins	1 oz.	120	10	4.0		T
Triscuit	1 oz.	120	20	4.0		T
Whole wheat						
Town House	1 oz.	140	6	2.0	♥	
Wheatables	1 oz.	140	18	3.0		
Zwieback toast	1 oz.	120	20	2.0	♥	
Crispbreads						
Crisp & Light	1 piece	17	3	0.0	♥	T
Ryvita	1 piece	23	4	0.4	♥	T
Wasa Breakfast	1 piece	50	8	1.0	♥	T
Wasa Extra Crisp	1 piece	25	5	0.0	♥	T
Wasa Fiber Plus	1 piece	35	5	1.0		T
Croissants	1	235	27	12.0		
Croutons						
cheese	1 oz.	140	13	9.0		
onion garlic	1 oz.	130	16	6.0		
plain	1 oz.	140	20	5.0		
seasoned	1 oz.	140	19	5.0		
English muffins						
cinnamon/raisin (Thomas')	1	140	27	2.0	♥	T
plain (Thomas')	1	130	27	1.0	♥	
raisin bran	1	150	28	3.0		T
Flour						
buckwheat	1 cup	340	78	1.0	♥	

♥ = HEALTHY HEART FOOD   T = TRIGGER FOOD

Item	SERVING	CAL-ORIES	CARBS (g)	TOTAL FAT(g)	♥	T
soy						
defatted	1 cup	330	40	1.2	♥	
full fat	1 cup	375	29	19.0		
low-fat	1 cup	285	33	2.4	♥	
white						
cake or pastry, sifted	1 cup	350	76	1.0	♥	
self-rising, unsifted	1 cup	440	93	1.0	♥	
sifted	1 cup	420	88	1.0	♥	
unsifted	1 cup	455	95	1.0	♥	
whole wheat	1 cup	400	85	2.0	♥	
French toast	1 slice	155	17	7.0		
Matzo						
egg	1 oz.	110	23	1.7	♥	
plain	1 oz.	110	24	0.3	♥	
Melba Toast						
bran	1 oz.	104	20	1.8	♥	T
plain	1 oz.	106	22	1.2	♥	T
rye	1 oz.	106	21	1.2	♥	T
Muffins						
blueberry						
commercial	1	120	23	3.0		
homemade	1	112	17	3.7		
bran-date	1	104	17	3.9		T
cinnamon apple	1	140	27	2.0	♥	
English muffins						
cinnamon/raisin (Thomas')	1	140	27	2.0	♥	T
plain (Thomas')	1	130	27	1.0	♥	
raisin bran	1	150	28	3.0		T
Pancakes						
buckwheat	1	55	6	2.0		
buttermilk	1	47	10	0.0	♥	
plain						
from batter, Aunt Jemima	1 waffle	71	14	0.5	♥	
from mix	1	60	8	2.0		
homemade	1	60	9	2.0		
whole wheat	1	36	8	0.2	♥	
Rolls						
cloverleaf	1	84	15	1.6	♥	
crescent	1	95	13	4.0		
dinner						
commercial	1	85	14	2.0		
homemade	1	120	20	3.0		
frankfurter	1	115	20	2.0	♥	

♥ = HEALTHY HEART FOOD   T = TRIGGER FOOD

Item	SERVING	CAL-ORIES	CARBS (g)	TOTAL FAT(g)	♥	T
hamburger	1	115	20	2.0	♥	
hard roll	1	156	30	1.6	♥	
hoagie	1	400	72	8.0		
kaiser	1	156	30	1.6	♥	
Parker House	1	57	9	1.7		
submarine	1	400	72	8.0		
Stuffing						
beef (Stove Top)	1 cup	360	42	18.0		
chicken (Stove Top)	1 cup	360	40	18.0		
cornbread (Stove Top)	1 cup	340	42	18.0		
herb (Stove Top)	1 cup	340	40	18.0		
pork (Stove Top)	1 cup	340	42	18.0		
turkey						
commercial (Stove Top)	1 cup	340	40	18.0		
homemade, dry	1 cup	500	50	31.0		
homemade, moist	1 cup	420	40	26.0		
Tortillas	1	65	13	1.0	♥	
Waffles						
blueberry						
frozen, Aunt Jemima	1	86	14	2.5		
frozen, Eggo	1	130	18	5.0		
buttermilk	1	86	14	2.5		
homestyle	1	120	17	5.0		
plain						
from mix	1	205	27	8.0		
homemade	1	245	26	13.0		
strawberry	1	130	18	5.0		

CEREALS

Item	SERVING	CAL-ORIES	CARBS (g)	TOTAL FAT(g)	♥	T
Note: Values for cereals are listed below; add calories, carbohydrates, and fat for any regular or lower fat milk added.						
All-Bran	1 oz.	70	21	1.0	♥	T
All-Bran, extra fiber	1 oz.	50	22	1.0	♥	T
Alpha Bits	1 oz.	110	24	1.0	♥	
Apple Cinnamon Cheerios	1 oz.	110	22	2.0	♥	

♥ = HEALTHY HEART FOOD   T = TRIGGER FOOD

Item	SERVING	CAL-ORIES	CARBS (g)	TOTAL FAT(g)	♥	T
Apple Cinnamon Squares, Kellogg's	1 oz.	90	23	0.0	♥	
Apple Jacks	1 oz.	110	26	0.0	♥	
Apple Raisin Crisp	1 oz.	100	25	0.0	♥	
Arrowhead Crunch	1 oz.	120	18	3.0		
Arrowhead Mills Instant	1 oz.	130	23	3.0		
Blueberry Squares, Kellogg's	1 oz.	90	23	0.0	♥	
Booberry	1 oz.	110	24	1.0	♥	
Bran Buds	1 oz.	70	22	1.0	♥	T
Bran Chex	1 oz.	90	24	0.0	♥	T
Bran Flakes, Arrowhead Mills	1 oz.	100	20	1.0	♥	T
Bran Flakes, Post Natural	1 oz.	90	23	0.0	♥	T
Cap'n Crunch	1 oz.	120	23	3.0		
Cap'n Crunch's Cruchberries	1 oz.	113	24	1.7	♥	
Cap'n Crunch's Peanut Butter	1 oz.	119	22	3.0		
Cheerios	1 oz.	110	20	2.0	♥	T
Cheerios, Apple Cinnamon	1 oz.	110	22	2.0	♥	
Cheerios, Honey Nut	1 oz.	110	23	1.0	♥	
Cinnamon Life	1 oz.	101	19	1.7	♥	
Cinnamon Toast Crunch	1 oz.	120	22	3.0		
Cocoa Crispies	1 oz.	110	25	0.0	♥	
Cocoa Pebbles	1 oz.	110	25	2.0	♥	
Cocoa Puffs	1 oz.	110	25	1.0	♥	
Common Sense w/raisins	1 oz.	92	22	0.0	♥	T
Cookie Crisp	1 oz.	110	25	1.0	♥	
Corn Bran	1 oz.	110	24	1.0	♥	
Corn Chex	1 oz.	110	25	0.0	♥	
Corn Flakes						
Health Valley	1 oz.	90	19	2.0		T
Kellogg's	1 oz.	110	24	0.0	♥	T
Total	1 oz.	110	24	0.0	♥	T
Corn grits						
instant	1 pkt.	80	18	0.0	♥	
quick	1 cup	145	31	0.0	♥	
regular	1 cup	145	31	0.0	♥	
Corn Pops	1 oz.	110	26	0.0	♥	
Count Chocula	1 oz.	110	24	1.0	♥	
Cracklin' Bran	1 oz.	120	20	4.0		
Cracklin' Oat Bran	1 oz.	110	20	0.0	♥	
Crisp Rice, Featherweight	1 oz.	110	26	0.0	♥	
Crispy Wheats 'n Raisins	1 oz.	110	23	1.0	♥	
Cream of Wheat						
instant	1 cup	140	29	0.0	♥	T
Mix'n Eat	1 pkt.	100	21	0.0	♥	T

♥ = HEALTHY HEART FOOD   T = TRIGGER FOOD

Item	SERVING	CAL-ORIES	CARBS (g)	TOTAL FAT(g)	♥	T
quick	1 cup	140	29	0.0	♥	T
regular	1 cup	140	29	0.0	♥	T
Crispix	1 oz.	110	22	0.0	♥	
Cruchberries, Cap'n Crunch	1 oz.	113	24	1.7	♥	
Crunchy Bran, Quaker	1 oz.	89	23	1.3	♥	
Crunchy Nut Oh's	1 oz.	127	22	4.2	♥	
Dinersaurs, Ralston	1 oz.	110	25	1.0	♥	
Farina, H-O Instant	1 pkt.	110	22	0.0	♥	
Farina, creamy, H-O	1 oz.	120	26	0.0	♥	
40% Bran Flakes						
Kellogg's	1 oz.	90	22	1.0	♥	T
Post	1 oz.	90	22	0.0	♥	T
Four Grain, Arrowhead Mills	1 oz.	94	18	1.0	♥	T
Froot Loops	1 oz.	110	25	1.0	♥	
Frosted Flakes, Kellogg's	1 oz.	110	26	0.0	♥	
Frosted Krispies, Kellogg's	1 oz.	110	26	0.0	♥	
Frosted Mini-Wheats	1 oz.	110	23	0.0	♥	
Fruit and Fiber	1 oz.	96	21	1.6	♥	T
Fruit & Fitness, Health Valley	1 oz.	95	16	1.5	♥	T
Fruit Lites, Health Valley	1 oz.	90	22	0.0	♥	
Fruit Muesli, Ralston	1 oz.	103	21	2.1	♥	T
Fruitful Bran	1 oz.	85	22	0.0	♥	T
Fruity Marshmallow, Krispies	1 oz.	108	25	0.0	♥	
Fruity Pebbles	1 oz.	110	25	1.0	♥	
Golden Grahams	1 oz.	110	24	1.0	♥	
Granola						
cinnamon-raisin, Nature Valley	1 oz.	130	19	5.0		T
regular, Nature Valley	1 oz.	130	19	5.0		T
w/almonds, Sun Country	1 oz.	130	19	5.3		T
w/banana & almonds, Sunbelt	1 oz.	120	19	5.0		
w/coconut & honey, Nature Valley	1 oz.	150	18	7.0		
w/fruit & nuts, Nature Valley	1 oz.	130	20	4.0		
w/fruit & nuts, Sunbelt	1 oz.	120	19	5.0		
w/raisins, Sun Country	1 oz.	125	19	4.8		
Grape-Nuts	1 oz.	100	23	0.0	♥	T
Grape-Nuts Flakes	1 oz.	110	23	0.0	♥	T
Health Valley Flakes	1 oz.	100	20	0.4	♥	
Health Valley Flakes, w/raisins	1 oz.	100	21	1.0	♥	
Healthy Crunch w/apple & cinnamon	1 oz.	100	16	3.0		T

♥ = HEALTHY HEART FOOD   T = TRIGGER FOOD

Item	SERVING	CAL-ORIES	CARBS (g)	TOTAL FAT(g)	♥	T
Heartland	1 oz.	120	18	4.0		T
Heartland w/coconut	1 oz.	130	18	5.0		T
Heartwise, Kellogg's	1 oz.	90	23	1.0	♥	T
Hominy grits						
instant	1 pkt.	80	18	0.0	♥	
quick	1 cup	145	31	0.0	♥	
regular	1 cup	145	31	0.0	♥	
Honey Bran	1 oz.	100	20	1.0	♥	
Honey Bunches of Oats	1 oz.	110	24	2.0	♥	
Honeycomb	1 oz.	110	25	0.0	♥	
Honey Graham Chex	1 oz.	110	25	1.0	♥	
Honey Graham Oh's	1 oz.	122	23	1.5	♥	
Honey Nut Cheerios	1 oz.	110	23	1.0	♥	
Honey & Nut Crunch Biscuits	1 oz.	100	22	1.0	♥	
Honey Smacks	1 oz.	110	25	1.0	♥	
Kix	1 oz.	110	24	1.0	♥	
Life	1 oz.	110	19	1.0	♥	T
Life, Cinnamon	1 oz.	110	19	1.0	♥	
Lucky Charms	1 oz.	110	23	1.0	♥	
Malt-O-Meal	1 cup	120	26	0.0	♥	
Muesli, Ralston	1 oz.	97	22	1.4	♥	
Muesli w/fruit, Ralston	1 oz.	103	21	2.1	♥	T
Mueslix	1 oz.	100	23	1.4	♥	T
Nutri-Grain	1 oz.	100	24	0.0	♥	T
Nutri-Grain Nuggets	1 oz.	100	23	1.0	♥	
Nutri-Grain, w/nuts & fruit	1 oz.	100	22	1.4	♥	
Nutri-Grain w/raisins	1 oz.	93	23	0.0	♥	T
Oat Bran w/raisins, General Mills	1 oz.	100	21	1.3	♥	
Oat Flakes	1 oz.	100	20	1.0	♥	
Oatmeal						
instant, flavored	1 pkt.	160	31	2.0	♥	
instant, H-O	1 pkt.	110	18	2.0	♥	T
instant, plain	1 pkt.	105	18	2.0	♥	T
instant, w/brown sugar, H-O	1 pkt.	152	32	2.1	♥	
instant w/spice, Quaker	1 pkt.	149	32	2.0	♥	
quick, H-O	1 pkt.	130	23	2.0	♥	
regular	1 cup	145	25	2.0	♥	T
Oatmeal Crisp	1 oz.	110	22	2.0	♥	
100% Bran	1 oz.	70	21	2.0		T
100% Bran, Nabisco	1 oz.	70	22	2.0		T
100% Natural Cereal	1 oz.	135	18	6.0		
100% Natural, Health Valley	1 oz.	70	22	1.0	♥	

♥ = HEALTHY HEART FOOD   T = TRIGGER FOOD

Item	SERVING	CAL-ORIES	CARBS (g)	TOTAL FAT(g)	♥	T
100% Natural, Nature Valley	1 oz.	120	20	4.0		
100% Natural, Quaker	1 oz.	126	19	4.9		T
100% Natural, Sun Country	1 oz.	123	20	4.5		
Product 19	1 oz.	110	24	0.0	♥	
Puffed Rice, Quaker	1 oz.	108	25	0.2	♥	T
Puffed Wheat						
Arrowhead Mills	1 oz.	100	22	0.0	♥	
Quaker	1 oz.	100	21	0.4	♥	T
Raisin Bran						
Kellogg's	1 oz.	90	21	1.0	♥	
Post	1 oz.	85	21	1.0	♥	
Total	1 oz.	93	22	0.7	♥	T
Raisin Nut Bran	1 oz.	110	20	3.0		
Raisin Oat Bran, General Mills	1 oz.	100	21	1.3	♥	
Raisin Squares, Kellogg's	1 oz.	90	23	0.0	♥	
Rice Bran, Health Valley	1 oz.	110	22	1.0	♥	
Rice Bran w/almonds & dates	1 oz.	110	19	3.0		
Rice Chex	1 oz.	110	25	0.0	♥	
Rice Krispies	1 oz.	110	25	0.0	♥	
Rolled Oats (see Oatmeal)						
Seven Grain, Arrowhead Mills	1 oz.	100	17	1.0	♥	
Shredded Wheat						
Nabisco	1 oz.	96	23	1.0	♥	T
Nutri-Grain	1 oz.	90	22	0.0	♥	
Quaker	1 oz.	94	23	0.4	♥	T
Shredded Wheat' n Bran, Nabisco	1 oz.	90	23	0.8	♥	
Smurf-Magic Berries	1 oz.	120	26	1.0	♥	
Special K	1 oz.	110	21	0.0	♥	T
Sugar Smacks	1 oz.	105	25	1.0	♥	
Super Golden Crisps	1 oz.	110	26	0.0	♥	
Super Sugar Crisp	1 oz.	105	26	0.0	♥	
Toasties, Post	1 oz.	110	24	0.0	♥	
Total	1 oz.	100	22	1.0	♥	
Total Quick	1 oz.	90	18	2.0		T
Trix	1 oz.	110	25	0.0	♥	
Wheat Chex	1 oz.	100	23	0.0	♥	
Wheat Flakes	1 oz.	110	23	1.0	♥	
Wheatena	1 oz.	100	21	1.0	♥	
Wheaties	1 oz.	100	23	0.0	♥	

♥ = HEALTHY HEART FOOD   T = TRIGGER FOOD

Item	SERVING	CAL-ORIES	CARBS (g)	TOTAL FAT(g)	♥	T
Note: Portions for combined canned or frozen foods are given in typical packaged amounts.						
Beef pot pie						
homemade	7 oz.	515	39	30.0		
Morton	7 oz.	430	27	31.0		
Beef stew						
Dinty Moore	8 oz.	210	16	11.0		
homemade	8 oz.	220	15	11.0		
Libby's	8 oz.	170	19	6.0		
Chicken a la king	1 cup	470	12	34.0		
Chicken & noodles	1 cup	365	26	18.0		
Chicken chow mein						
canned	1 cup	95	18	0.0		T
homemade	1 cup	255	10	10.0		T
Chicken chow mein entree, La Choy	¾ cup	80	8	3.0		T
Chicken chow mein oriental, La Choy	¾ cup	240	47	2.0	♥	T
Chicken pot pie						
Banquet	7 oz.	550	39	36.0		
homemade	7 oz.	545	42	31.0		
Swanson	7 oz.	370	35	22.0		
Chicken salad (3 oz. scoop)						
commercial	1 scoop	192	9	15.0		T
homemade	1 scoop	190	1	15.0		
Chili con carne w/beans	8 oz.	340	31	16.0		
Chili w/beans, canned						
Dennison's	8 oz.	340	29	17.0		
Hormel	8 oz.	320	25	17.0		
Chili w/o beans, canned						
Dennison's	8 oz.	320	15	20.2		
Hormel	8 oz.	413	12	31.7		
Chop suey	1 cup	300	13	17.0		T
Corned Beef Hash, canned						
Libby's	8 oz.	420	21	28.0		
Mary Kitchen	8 oz.	427	20	25.6		
Egg roll						
chicken	1 roll	220	32	8.0		T
pork	1 roll	180	23	6.0		T
vegetarian	1 roll	160	20	6.0		T
French bread pizza w/pepperoni	4½ oz.	350	36	16.0		T

♥ = HEALTHY HEART FOOD   T = TRIGGER FOOD

Item	SERVING	CAL-ORIES	CARBS (g)	TOTAL FAT(g)	♥	T
French Toast Breakfast, cinnamon swirls w/sausage	5½ oz.	390	37	21.0		
Fried rice						
w/chicken	8 oz.	260	41	4.0		T
w/pork	8 oz.	270	44	6.0	♥	T
Frozen Meals						
Beef, Oriental	10 oz.	290	36	9.0		
Beef Stroganoff	10 oz.	430	28	24.0		
Chicken, dark meat	9¾ oz.	560	55	28.0		
Chicken, Hungry Man	17¾ oz.	700	65	28.0		
Chicken, Mesquite	10½ oz.	310	52	2.0	♥	
Chicken, sweet & sour						
Healthy Choice	11½ oz.	280	44	2.0	♥	T
Le Menu	11¼ oz.	400	41	18.0		
Tyson Gourmet	11 oz.	420	50	15.0		
Chicken a la King	12 oz.	320	37	8.0		
Chicken cacciatore	11 oz.	300	27	13.0		
Chicken chow mein	13 oz.	370	53	6.0		T
Chicken in herb cream	9½ oz.	260	17	10.0		
Chicken Kiev	8 oz.	530	24	39.0		
Chicken Marsala	10½ oz.	300	26	13.0		
Chicken Oriental	10¾ oz.	270	32	7.0		
Chicken Parmigiana						
Celantano	9 oz.	330	15	20.0		
Healthy Choice	11½ oz.	280	38	3.0	♥	T
Tyson Gourmet	11¼ oz.	380	37	17.0		
Chopped sirloin	10¾ oz.	340	28	16.0		
Egg substitute breakfast						
w/hash browns & links	7 oz.	360	22	23.0		
w/pancakes & links	6.8 oz.	380	33	19.0		
Enchilada						
beef	12 oz.	500	72	15.0		
cheese	12 oz.	550	71	19.0		
chicken	11 oz.	460	54	18.0		
Fajita, beef	12 oz.	500	62	14.0		
Fettuccini Alfredo	12 oz.	360	54	13.0		
Fettuccini w/meat sauce	12 oz.	348	41	12.0		
Fish & Chips	12 oz.	600	72	25.2		
Fried chicken	10 oz.	400	45	22.0		
Ham steak	10 oz.	400	43	17.0		
Lasagna, Banquet Extra	16½ oz.	645	88	23.0		
Macaroni & beef	12 oz.	370	48	15.0		
Macaroni & cheese	10 oz.	420	46	20.0		
Manicotti, three cheese	11¾ oz.	390	44	15.0		

♥ = HEALTHY HEART FOOD   T = TRIGGER FOOD

Item	SERVING	CAL-ORIES	CARBS (g)	TOTAL FAT(g)	♥	T
Meat loaf						
Banquet	11 oz.	440	27	27.0		
Morton	10 oz.	310	26	17.0		
Swanson	10¾ oz.	360	41	15.0		
Meatball	11¼ oz.	330	23	18.0		
Meatball stew	8 oz.	240	15	15.0		
Noodle & Chicken	10 oz.	350	42	15.0		
Pasta shells & beef	8 oz.	272	27	11.2		
Pepper steak, Healthy Choice	9½ oz.	250	36	4.0	♥	
Pork loin	10¾ oz.	280	27	12.0		
Roast beef	9½ oz.	330	36	14.0		
Roast beef, Hungry Man	16¾ oz.	640	41	37.0		
Roast beef, Swanson	11¼ oz.	310	38	6.0		
Salisbury steak						
Banquet	11 oz.	500	26	34.0		
Swanson	10¾ oz.	400	43	17.0		
Shrimp, Healthy Choice	11¼ oz.	210	42	1.0	♥	T
Spaghetti w/meat balls	10 oz.	290	44	10.0		
Tortellini w/meat	10 oz.	250	8	10.0		
Turkey	10½ oz.	390	35	20.0		
Turkey, Hungry Man	17 oz.	550	61	18.0		
Turkey breast, Healthy Choice	10½ oz.	290	39	5.0	♥	T
Veal Marsala, Le Menu Light	10 oz.	230	28	3.0	♥	T
Veal Parmigiana						
Hungry Man	18¼ oz.	590	57	26.0		
Le Menu	11½ oz.	390	36	17.0		
Welsh rarebit	10 oz.	350	8	30.0		
Green pepper stuffed w/beef	7½ oz.	200	19	9.0		
Ham and cheese pocket, frozen	5 oz.	360	36	16.0		
Linguine w/scallops & clams	9½ oz.	280	28	11.0		
Linguine w/shrimp	10 oz.	330	33	15.0		
Lobster Newburg	6½ oz.	380	9	32.0		
Macaroni & cheese						
canned	1 cup	230	26	10.0		
homemade	1 cup	430	40	22.0		
Macaroni w/beef						
Chef Boyardee Beefaroni	7½ oz.	220	31	7.0		
Franco-American	7½ oz.	170	24	6.0		
Pasta w/chicken & herbs	½ cup	170	21	7.0		
Pasta w/meatballs						
Buitoni Rings or twists	7½ oz.	210	28	7.0		

♥ = HEALTHY HEART FOOD   T = TRIGGER FOOD

Item	SERVING	CAL-ORIES	CARBS (g)	TOTAL FAT(g)	♥	T
Chef Boyardee Dinosaurs	8 oz.	256	34	9.6		
Franco American Teddy O's	8 oz.	224	27	8.5		
Lipton Hearty Ones	11 oz.	328	63	1.9		
Pizza pocket sandwich w/sausage	5 oz.	360	40	16.0		
Pizza, frozen						
w/cheese	¼ pie	317	28	16.6		
w/cheese & pepperoni, vegetable	¼ pie	380	34	18.0		
Celeste	¼ pie	310	28	16.0		T
Celeste Pizza for One	1 pie	490	44	26.0		T
Veg Deluxe, Stouffer's	½ pkg	420	41	20.0		T
Pizza, french bread w/pepperoni	4½ oz.	350	36	16.0		
Quiche Lorraine	⅛ quiche	600	29	48.0		
Ravioli, beef w/meat sauce						
Buitoni	7½ oz.	180	28	4.0		
RavioliO's	7½ oz.	250	35	8.0		
Shrimp cocktail, Sau-Sea	4 oz.	113	19	1.0	♥	T
Shrimp salad (3 oz. scoop)						
commercial	1 scoop	126	6	9.0		T
homemade	1 scoop	128	1	9.0		
Spaghetti w/beef	7½ oz.	220	27	9.0		
Spaghetti w/meatballs						
Buitoni	7½ oz.	190	21	8.0		
homemade	1 cup	330	39	12.0		
SpaghettiOs	7½ oz.	220	28	8.0		
Spaghetti w/tomato sauce & cheese						
canned	1 cup	190	39	2.0	♥	
homemade	1 cup	260	37	9.0		
Tuna salad (3 oz. scoop)						
commercial	1 scoop	174	9	12.0		T
homemade	1 scoop	170	1	11.0		

DAIRY

Item	SERVING	CAL-ORIES	CARBS (g)	TOTAL FAT(g)	♥	T
Butter and butter substitutes, see our Fats & Oils section.						
Cheese						
blue	1 oz.	100	1	8.0		

♥ = HEALTHY HEART FOOD   T = TRIGGER FOOD

Item	SERVING	CAL-ORIES	CARBS (g)	TOTAL FAT(g)	♥	T
Brie	1 oz.	95	0	7.9		
Brie, Dorman's	1 oz.	81	0	6.6		
Camembert	1 oz.	86	0	6.8		
cheddar	1 oz.	115	0	9.0		
Colby	1 oz.	112	1	9.1		
cottage cheese						
large curd	1 oz.	57	1	1.2		T
low-fat	1 oz.	26	1	0.5	♥	T
small curd	1 oz.	27	1	1.1		T
uncreamed	1 oz.	16	0	0.1	♥	T
w/fruit	1 oz.	35	4	1.0		T
cream cheese						
light (Neufchatel)	1 oz.	80	1	7.0		
most brands	1 oz.	100	1	10.0		
soft	1 oz.	100	2	9.0		
w/chives	1 oz.	90	1	8.0		
w/onions	1 oz.	90	2	8.0		
Edam	1 oz.	101	0	7.9		
farmer	1 oz.	40	1	3.0		
feta	1 oz.	75	1	6.0		
Gouda	1 oz.	101	1	7.8		
Havarti						
Dorman's 60%	1 oz.	118	0	10.6		
most brands	1 oz.	120	0	11.0		
Jarlsberg	1 oz.	100	1	7.0		
Limburger	1 oz.	93	0	7.7		
Monterey Jack	1 oz.	106	0	8.6		
mozzarella						
part skim	1 oz.	70	1	4.0		
whole milk	1 oz.	90	1	7.0		
muenster						
Crowley	1 oz.	90	1	7.0		
Dorman's	1 oz.	110	0	9.0		
most brands	1 oz.	105	0	9.0		
Parmesan, grated	1 oz.	130	0	9.0		
provolone	1 oz.	100	1	8.0		
ricotta						
light, Polly-O	1 oz.	40	2	2.0		
low-fat, Frigo	1 oz.	20	1	1.0		
part skim milk	1 oz.	45	1	3.0		
whole milk	1 oz.	50	1	3.5		
Romano	1 oz.	110	1	7.6		
Roquefort	1 oz.	105	1	8.7		
string	1 oz.	80	1	5.0		

♥ = HEALTHY HEART FOOD   T = TRIGGER FOOD

Item	SERVING	CAL-ORIES	CARBS (g)	TOTAL FAT(g)	♥	T
Swiss	1 oz.	105	1	8.0		
Tilsit	1 oz.	100	1	7.0		
Cheese food						
American	1 oz.	95	2	7.0		T
American, processed	1 oz.	93	2	7.0		T
Swiss, processed	1 oz.	92	1	6.8		
Cheese spread						
American	1 oz.	80	2	6.0		T
Cheese substitutes						
cheddar, from tofu	1 oz.	80	1	8.0		
cheddar, Sargento	1 oz.	90	1	6.0		
colby, Dorman's LoChol	1 oz.	90	1	6.0		
cream cheese, Tofutti	1 oz.	80	1	8.0		
mozzarella, Sargento	1 oz.	80	1	6.0		
Muenster, Dorman's LoChol	1 oz.	100	1	7.0		
Swiss, Dorman's LoChol	1 oz.	100	1	7.0		
Cocoa						
w/low-fat milk powder	8 fl oz.	133	29	1.0	♥	
w/whole milk	8 fl oz.	225	30	9.0		
Cream						
half & half	1 Tbsp.	20	1	2.0		
heavy	1 Tbsp.	50	0	6.0		
ice cream, see our Sweets, Desserts, & Toppings section						
light	1 Tbsp.	30	1	3.0		
sour	1 Tbsp.	25	1	3.0		
whipped topping						
heavy	1 Tbsp.	52	0	5.6		
light	1 Tbsp.	44	0	4.6		
pressurized	1 Tbsp.	8	0	0.7		
Cream substitute (non-dairy)						
from frozen	1 tsp.	10	2	0.5		
liquid, Rich's Coffee Rich	1 tsp.	7	1	0.7		
powder						
Coffee-mate	1 tsp.	10	1	0.6		
Coffee-mate Lite	1 tsp.	8	2	0.5		
Cremora	1 tsp.	10	1	0.6		
sour cream	1 Tbsp.	25	1	2.0		
whipped topping						
frozen						
Cool Whip	1 Tbsp.	12	1	1.0		
Lite Cool Whip	1 Tbsp.	8	1	0.5		
most brands	1 Tbsp.	15	1	1.0		
pressurized	1 Tbsp.	10	1	1.0		

♥ = HEALTHY HEART FOOD   T = TRIGGER FOOD

Item	SERVING	CAL-ORIES	CARBS (g)	TOTAL FAT(g)	♥	T
Eggs						
fried in butter	1	95	1	7.0		
hard boiled	1	80	1	6.0		
poached	1	80	1	6.0		
scrambled w/milk & butter	1	110	2	8.0		
raw						
white part only	1	15	0	0.0	♥	
whole egg	1	80	1	6.0		
yolk only	1	65	0	6.0		
Egg substitutes						
frozen						
Egg Beaters, Fleischmann's	¼ cup	25	1	0.0	♥	
Egg Watchers, Tofutti	¼ cup	50	2	2.0		
Scramblers, Morningstar Farms	¼ cup	60	3	3.0		T
liquid	¼ cup	52	1	2.1		
mix						
Tofu Scrambler w/butter	¼ cup	79	4	6.0		T
Tofu Scrambler, w/o butter	¼ cup	49	4	2.5		T
Ice Cream, see our Sweets, Desserts, & Toppings section						
Malted Milk						
chocolate w/whole milk	8 fl oz.	85	18	10.0		
natural w/whole milk (also see Shakes)	8 fl oz.	235	27	10.0		
Milk						
buttermilk	8 fl oz.	100	12	2.0	♥	
chocolate, low-fat 1%	8 fl oz.	160	26	3.0	♥	
chocolate, low-fat 2%	8 fl oz.	180	26	5.0		
chocolate, regular	8 fl oz.	210	26	8.0		
condensed, sweetened	8 fl oz.	980	166	27.0		
dried, nonfat instant	8 fl oz.	245	35	0.0	♥	
evaporated, skim	8 fl oz.	200	29	1.0	♥	
evaporated, whole milk	8 fl oz.	340	25	19.0		
low-fat (1%)	8 fl oz.	100	12	3.0		T
low-fat (2%)	8 fl oz.	120	12	5.0		T
nonfat	8 fl oz.	85	12	0.0	♥	T
skim	8 fl oz.	85	12	0.0	♥	T
whole	8 fl oz.	150	11	8.0		T
Milk substitute						
from soy milk	8 fl oz.	79	4	4.6		
from vegetable oil	8 fl oz.	136	16	16.0		T

♥ = HEALTHY HEART FOOD   T = TRIGGER FOOD

Item	SERVING	CAL-ORIES	CARBS (g)	TOTAL FAT(g)	♥	T
Shakes						
chocolate, thick	8 fl oz.	268	48	6.4		
vanilla, thick	8 fl oz.	252	40	7.2		
Soy beverages						
carob, Ah Soy	8 fl oz.	213	40	4.0	♥	
Soy Moo	8 fl oz.	125	11	5.0		
vanilla, Ah Soy	8 fl oz.	213	31	6.7		
Soy milk	8 fl oz.	79	4	4.6		
Yogurt						
(for frozen yogurt—see our Sweets, Desserts, & Toppings section)						
flavored, Dannon vanilla/ coffee	8 oz.	200	34	3.0	♥	
plain, low-fat	8 oz.	145	16	4.0		T
plain, nonfat	8 oz.	125	17	0.0	♥	T
plain, whole milk	8 oz.	140	11	7.0		T
w/fruit, Colombo, most flavors	8 oz.	230	36	6.0		
w/fruit, Dannon, most flavors	8 oz.	240	43	3.0	♥	
w/fruit, w/milk solids	8 oz.	230	43	2.0	♥	

DINING OUT—ETHNIC STYLE

Item	SERVING	CAL-ORIES	CARBS (g)	TOTAL FAT(g)	♥	T
Delicatessen Dining						
Bagel						
cinnamon & raisin						
dry	1	300	55	2.0	♥	T
w/butter	1 w/1 Tbsp.	400	55	13.0		T
w/cr. cheese	1 w/1 oz.	400	58	12.0		T
w/margarine	1 w/1 Tbsp.	400	55	13.0		T
egg						
dry	1	250	54	3.0	♥	
w/butter	1 w/1 Tbsp.	350	54	14.0		
w/cream cheese	1 w/1 oz.	350	57	13.0		
w/margarine	1 w/1 Tbsp.	350	54	14.0		
garlic/onion						
dry	1	220	43	2.0	♥	

♥ = HEALTHY HEART FOOD   T = TRIGGER FOOD

Item	SERVING	CAL-ORIES	CARBS (g)	TOTAL FAT(g)	♥	T
w/butter	1 w/1 Tbsp.	320	43	13.0		
w/cream cheese	1 w/1 oz.	320	46	12.0		
w/margarine	1 w/1 Tbsp.	320	43	13.0		
plain						
dry	1	200	38	2.0	♥	T
w/butter	1 w/1 Tbsp.	300	38	13.0		T
w/cream cheese	1 w/1 oz.	300	41	12.0		T
w/margarine	1 w/1 Tbsp.	300	38	13.0		T
poppy seed						
dry	1	205	38	2.0	♥	
w/butter	1 w/1 Tbsp.	305	38	13.0		
w/cream cheese	1 w/1 oz.	305	41	12.0		
w/margarine	1 w/1 Tbsp.	305	38	13.0		
sesame seed						
dry	1	205	38	2.0	♥	
w/butter	1 w/1 Tbsp.	305	38	13.0		
w/cream cheese	1 w/1 oz.	305	41	12.0		
w/margarine	1 w/1 Tbsp.	305	38	13.0		
Bologna sandwich on rye	1	432	36	13.8		
Brisket sandwich on rye	1	510	24	30.0		
Chicken liver, chopped	½ cup	275	3	17.0		
Cole slaw	½ cup	42	8	1.6		T
Dill pickle	1 med.	11	2	0.1	♥	
Frankfurter w/bun	1	295	22	18.0		T
Gefilte fish						
jelly	1 piece	92	6	2.0	♥	T
natural	1 piece	50	4	1.0	♥	T
Ham sandwich on rye	1	352	32	6.2		
Hot dog w/bun	1	295	22	18.0		T
Knockwurst w/bun	1	475	22	34.0		T
Liver, chicken chopped	½ cup	275	3	17.0		
Pickle, dill	1 medium	11	2	0.1	♥	
Potato pancake, homestyle	1 large	495	26	12.6		
Potato salad	½ cup	350	32	22.0		
Pumpernickel	1 slice	80	16	1.0	♥	
Roast beef sandwich on rye	1	567	24	37.8		
Roll, frankfurter	1	115	20	2.0	♥	
Rye bread						
plain	1 slice	65	12	1.0	♥	
w/seeds	1 slice	76	16	0.9	♥	
Salami sandwich on rye	1	450	27	30.0		
Sauerkraut	½ cup	22	5	0.2	♥	
Tongue on rye	1	381	24	19.6		
Turkey breast sandwich	1	272	36	5.8		

♥ = HEALTHY HEART FOOD   T = TRIGGER FOOD

Item	SERVING	CAL-ORIES	CARBS (g)	TOTAL FAT(g)	♥	T
French Dining						
Beef Burgundy	1 serv.	350	6	29.5		
Cheesecake, strawberry	1 slice	240	28	13.0		
Chicken Cordon Bleu	1 serv.	390	11	29.8		
Crepe						
beef burgundy	1 serv.	620	40	34.0		
chicken	1 serv.	550	25	30.0		
mushroom	1 serv.	500	52	26.0		
spinach	1 serv.	520	38	32.0		
French bread	1 slice	100	18	1.0	♥	
Pâté						
chicken liver	1 oz.	26	1	1.7		
goose liver	1 oz.	60	1	5.7		
Quiche Lorraine	1 serv.	600	29	48.0		
Italian Dining						
Chicken cacciatore	8 oz.	245	30	7.3		
Chicken Florentine	8 oz.	270	31	8.2		
Chicken Marsala	8 oz.	266	38	5.7	♥	
Chicken Parmigiana	8 oz.	270	24	14.1		
Chicken Piccata	8 oz.	238	19	9.8		
Chicken primavera	8 oz.	220	16	2.6	♥	
Fettuccini Alfredo	8 oz.	280	15	13.0		
Fettuccini Alfredo w/shrimp	8 oz.	265	26	17.0		
Italian bread	1 slice	85	17	0.0	♥	
Lasagna	8 oz.	290	27	8.8		
Linguini w/scallops	8 oz.	270	25	9.3		
Linguini w/shrimp	8 oz.	278	26	12.2		
Manicotti	8 oz.	420	42	12.3		
Minestrone	8 oz.	175	26	3.4	♥	
Parmesan cheese	1 tbsp.	23	0	1.5		
Pasta marinara	8 oz.	360	65	3.2		
Pasta w/pesto	8 oz.	570	87	18.0		
Pasta primavera	8 oz.	420	60	16.2		
Pasta shells, stuffed	8 oz.	440	42	11.8		
Pizza						
w/cheese	1 slice	320	32	13.9		
w/cheese & pepperoni	1 slice	360	32	19.2		
Ravioli						
beef in beef & tomato sauce	8 oz.	290	37	11.9		
beef in tomato sauce	8 oz.	250	30	11.0		
cheese in tomato sauce	8 oz.	200	34	4.1		

♥ = HEALTHY HEART FOOD   T = TRIGGER FOOD

Item	SERVING	CAL-ORIES	CARBS (g)	TOTAL FAT(g)	♥	T
Rigatoni w/meat sauce & cheese	8 oz.	255	23	9.7		
Shrimp fettuccini Alfredo	8 oz.	265	26	17.0		
Spaghetti w/tomato sauce & cheese	1 serv.	520	74	18.0		
Spaghetti w/tomato sauce & meat balls	1 serv.	660	78	24.0		
Spaghetti dinner, w/tomato sauce, meat balls, & garlic bread	1 serv.	940	134	33.0		
Tortellini & vegetable soup	8 oz.	84	13	3.5		
Wine, table, red	3½ oz.	75	3	0.0		T
Wine, table, white	3½ oz.	80	3	0.0		T
Ziti in marinara sauce	1 serv.	220	25	9.0		
Zucchini, breaded	½ cup	200	24	10.0		
Zucchini, in tomato juice	½ cup	33	8	0.2	♥	T
Mexican Dining						
Beans, refried	1 serv.	331	79	6.0		
Burrito, beans w/sauce	1	355	53	10.5		
Burrito, beef & beans w/sauce	1	470	72	11.6		
Burrito, beef w/sauce	1	400	38	17.6		
Chili con carne w/beans	1 serv.	370	28	20.8		
Chimi	1 serv.	487	43	19.0		
Churro	1 serv.	122	12	7.0		
Enchilada						
beef	1	330	49	10.4		
cheese	1	345	48	13.2		
chicken	1	310	35	12.6		
Enchirito w/sauce	1	377	30	19.7		
Fajita, chicken	1	226	20	10.2		
Fajita, steak	1	234	20	10.9		
Nachos	1 serv.	346	38	18.5		
Picante sauce	1 Tbsp.	4	1	0.0	♥	
Plantain, cooked	1 serv.	89	24	0.1	♥	
Taco, regular	1	183	11	10.8		
Taco dip	2 Tbsp.	12	3	0.0	♥	
Taco salad w/salsa	1 serv.	380	40	15.0		
Taco sauce	2 Tbsp.	10	2	0.0	♥	
Taco shell	1	50	8	2.1		
Tamale dinner	1	450	52	20.0		
Tortilla, corn	1	65	13	1.0	♥	
Tortilla, wheat	1	80	14	2.0		
Tostada w/sauce	1 serv.	240	26	11.1		
Tostada shell	1	73	10	3.5		

♥ = HEALTHY HEART FOOD   T = TRIGGER FOOD

Item	SERVING	CAL-ORIES	CARBS (g)	TOTAL FAT(g)	♥	T
Middle-Eastern Dining						
Falafel	3 patties	270	22	15.0		T
Pita bread	1	165	33	1.0	♥	T
Tahini	1 Tbsp.	89	3	8.1		
Tempeh	1 oz.	56	5	2.2		
Oriental Dining						
Beef w/broccoli	1 serv.	390	55	8.1		T
Beef w/vegetables & rice	1 serv.	340	48	10.4		T
Beef teriyaki w/peppers & rice	1 serv.	335	66	12.0		T
Chicken, sweet & sour w/rice	1 serv.	460	66	9.4		T
Chicken teriyaki	1 serv.	355	19	6.8		T
Chop suey w/rice	1 serv.	350	37	8.0		T
Chop suey w/beef & pork	1 serv.	600	26	34.0		T
Chow mein w/beef	1 serv.	280	32	4.0		T
Chow mein w/chicken	1 serv.	320	32	12.0		T
Egg roll	1	180	23	6.2		T
Green pepper steak w/rice	1 serv.	335	42	12.4		T
Noodles						
Chinese chow mein	1 cup	237	26	13.8		T
Chow mein noodles	1 cup	220	26	11.0		T
Japanese soba, cooked	1 cup	113	24	0.1	♥	T
Japanese somen, cooked	1 cup	230	49	0.3	♥	T
Japanese Udon, cooked	1 cup	230	23	0.6	♥	T
Rice, brown	1 cup	230	50	1.0	♥	T
Rice, white	1 cup	225	50	0.0	♥	T
Tea, brewed	1 cup	0	0	0.0	♥	T
Teriyaki/soy sauce	1 Tbsp.	15	3	0.0	♥	
Won Ton soup	1 cup	120	5	2.0		T
Other Ethnic Dining Specialties						
Beef Stroganoff w/parsley noodles	1 serv.	475	32	26.0		
Cabbage, stuffed w/meat in sauce	1 cabbage	175	16	8.1		T
Chicken Kiev	1 serv.	530	24	41.1		
Kielbasa	1 serv.	390	4	30.0		T

♥ = HEALTHY HEART FOOD   T = TRIGGER FOOD

Item	SERVING	CAL-ORIES	CARBS (g)	TOTAL FAT(g)	♥	T
Arby's						
Beef 'n cheddar sandwich	1	455	28	26.8		
Chicken breast sandwich	1	493	48	25.0		
French fries	1 order	246	30	13.2		
Ham 'n cheese sandwich	1	292	19	13.7		
Roast beef sandwich, regular	1	353	32	14.8		
Roast beef sandwich, super	1	501	50	22.1		
Roast chicken club sandwich	1	610	40	33.0		
Shake						
chocolate	1	384	50	11.5		
vanilla	1	350	46	10.0		
Turkey deluxe sandwich	1	375	33	16.6		
Arthur Treachers						
Chicken	1 order	369	17	21.6		
Chicken sandwich	1	413	44	19.2		
Chips (french fries)	1 order	276	35	13.2		
Cole slaw	1 order	123	11	8.2		T
Fish	1 order	355	25	19.8		
Fish sandwich	1	440	39	24.0		
Krunch Pup	1	203	12	14.8		
Shrimp	1 order	381	27	24.4		
Brazier—See Dairy Queen						
Burger King						
Bacon double cheeseburger	1	515	26	31.0		
Bagel						
plain	1	272	44	6.0		T
w/bacon, egg & cheese	1	453	46	20.0		
w/cream cheese	1	370	25	16.0		T
w/egg & cheese	1	407	46	16.0		
w/ham, egg, & cheese	1	438	46	17.0		
w/sausage, egg, & cheese	1	626	49	36.0		
Biscuit						
w/bacon & egg	1	568	45	36.0		
w/sausage & egg	1	568	35	36.0		
Catfish fillet	1	495	49	25.0		
Cheeseburger						
deluxe	1	390	29	23.0		
double cheeseburger	1	483	29	27.0		
double w/bacon	1	515	26	31.0		
regular	1	318	28	15.0		

♥ = HEALTHY HEART FOOD   T = TRIGGER FOOD

Item	SERVING	CAL-ORIES	CARBS (g)	TOTAL FAT(g)	♥	T
(also see Hamburgers)						
Chicken sandwich	1	685	56	40.0		
Chicken tenders	1 order	236	14	13.0		
Croissan'wich						
w/bacon, egg, & cheese	1	361	19	24.0		
w/egg & cheese	1	315	19	20.0		
w/ham egg & cheese	1	346	19	21.0		
w/sausage, egg, & cheese	1	534	22	40.0		
Danish						
apple cinnamon	1	390	62	13.0		
cheese	1	406	60	16.0		
Cheeseburger, double	1	483	29	27.0		
Eggs, see Scrambled eggs						
French toast sticks	1 serv.	538	53	32.0		
Hamburgers						
deluxe	1	344	28	19.0		
regular	1	272	28	11.0		
(also see Whopper)						
Mini muffin						
blueberry	1	292	37	14.0		
raisin oat bran	1	291	46	12.0		T
Salads						
chef salad w/o dressing	1	170	7	9.0		T
chunky chicken w/o dressing	1	142	8	4.0		T
garden w/o dressing	1	95	8	5.0		T
side salad w/o dressing	1	25	5	0.0	♥	T
Scrambled eggs	1 order	549	44	34.0		
Scrambled eggs w/bacon	1 order	610	44	34.0		
Scrambled eggs w/sausage	1 order	768	47	53.0		
Whopper	1	614	45	36.0		
Whopper deluxe w/cheese	1	935	47	61.0		
Whopper double	1	844	45	53.0		
Whopper w/cheese	1	706	47	44.0		
Carls Jr						
Bacon, side order	2 strips	50	0	4.0		
Roast Beef'n Swiss	1	360	43	8.0		
Charbroiler BBQ Chicken	1	320	40	5.0	♥	
Charbroiler Chicken Club	1	510	53	22.0		
Cheeseburger, Western Bacon	1	630	49	33.0		
(also see Hamburgers)						
Country Fried Steak	1	610	54	33.0		

♥ = HEALTHY HEART FOOD   T = TRIGGER FOOD

Item	SERVING	CAL-ORIES	CARBS (g)	TOTAL FAT(g)	♥	T
Danish	1	519	73	21.0		
Fish fillet	1	550	58	26.0		
French fries	1 order	360	43	17.0		
French toast dips w/o syrup	1 serv.	180	28	6.0		
Hamburgers,						
Famous Star	1	360	43	8.0		
Happy Star	1	220	26	8.0		
Old Time Star	1	400	38	17.0		
Super Star	1	770	44	50.0		
Hash brown nuggets	1 serv.	170	20	9.0		
Hotcakes w/o syrup	1 serv.	360	59	12.0		
Muffin						
blueberry	1	256	40	7.0		
bran	1	220	34	6.0		T
Onion rings	1 order	310	38	15.0		
Potato						
w/bacon & cheese	1	650	63	34.0		
w/broccoli & cheese	1	470	61	17.0		
Lite	1	250	54	3.0	♥	T
Salads						
Chef Salad-to-go	1	180	11	7.0		T
Chicken Salad-to-go	1	206	12	8.0		T
Garden Salad-to-go	1	46	4	2.0		
Sausage patties	1	190	1	17.0		
Scrambled eggs	1 order	120	2	9.0		
Shakes						
chocolate	1	353	61	7.0		
vanilla	1	353	61	7.0		
Soups						
Boston clam chowder	1 order	140	12	8.0		
chicken noodle soup	1 order	80	11	1.0	♥	
cream of broccoli soup	1 order	140	14	6.0		
vegetable soup	1 order	70	10	3.0		T
Sunrise sandwich						
w/bacon	1	370	32	19.0		
w/sausage	1	500	31	32.0		
Zucchini	1 order	300	33	16.0		
Dairy Queen/Brazier						
BBQ Beef	1	225	34	4.0		
Chicken fillet						
breaded	1	430	37	20.0		
breaded w/cheese	1	480	38	25.0		
grilled	1	300	33	8.0		

♥ = HEALTHY HEART FOOD   T = TRIGGER FOOD

Item	SERVING	CAL-ORIES	CARBS (g)	TOTAL FAT(g)	♥	T
Cheeseburger, see Hamburgers						
Fish fillet						
regular	1	370	39	16.0		
w/cheese	1	420	40	21.0		
French fries, regular	1 order	300	40	14.0		
Hamburgers						
double	1	460	29	25.0		
double w/cheese	1	570	31	34.0		
single	1	310	29	13.0		
single w/cheese	1	365	30	18.0		
Homestyle Ultimate Burger	1	700	30	47.0		
Hot Dogs						
regular	1	280	23	16.0		T
w/cheese	1	330	24	21.0		
w/chili	1	320	26	19.0		
Super Dog	1	590	41	38.0		
Ice cream						
Big Scoop, chocolate	1 order	310	40	14.0		
Big Scoop, vanilla	1 order	300	39	14.0		
Buster bar	1	450	40	29.0		
Cone, chocolate	1	230	36	7.0		
Cone, vanilla	1	230	36	7.0		
Dilly Bar	1	210	21	13.0		
Sandwich	1	140	24	4.0		
Mr. Misty	1 regular	250	63	0.0	♥	
Onion rings, regular	1 order	240	29	12.0		
Shake						
Blizzard, Heath, regular	1	820	114	36.0		
Blizzard, Strawberry, regular	1	740	92	16.0		
Breeze, Heath, regular	1	680	113	21.0		
chocolate, regular	1	540	94	14.0		
malted, regular	1	610	106	14.0		
vanilla, regular	1	520	88	14.0		
Breeze, Strawberry, regular	1	590	90	10.0		
Yogurt (frozen), regular cone	1	180	38	0.6	♥	T
Yogurt (frozen), regular cup	1	170	35	0.6	♥	T
Domino's Pizza						
Pizzas (16")						
Cheese	1 slice	188	28	5.1		
Deluxe	1 slice	249	30	10.2		
Double cheese w/pepperoni	1 slice	273	28	12.7		

♥ = HEALTHY HEART FOOD   T = TRIGGER FOOD

Item	SERVING	CAL-ORIES	CARBS (g)	TOTAL FAT(g)	♥	T
Ham	1 slice	209	29	5.5		
Pepperoni	1 slice	230	28	8.8		
Sausage w/mushroom	1 slice	215	28	7.9		
Vegetable pizza	1 slice	249	30	9.3		T
Hardee's						
Big Country Brekfast						
w/bacon	1 order	660	51	40.0		
w/ham	1 order	620	51	33.0		
w/sausage	1 order	850	51	57.0		
Big Twin	1 order	450	34	25.0		
Biscuits						
bacon	1	360	34	21.0		
bacon & egg	1	410	35	24.0		
bacon, egg, & cheese	1	460	35	28.0		
Biscuit 'N' Gravy	1	440	45	24.0		
Canadian Rise 'N' Shine	1	470	35	27.0		
chicken	1	430	42	22.0		
Cinnamon 'N' Raisin	1	320	37	17.0		
country ham	1	350	35	18.0		
country ham & egg	1	370	35	19.0		
ham	1	320	34	16.0		
ham & egg	1	370	35	19.0		
ham, egg, & cheese	1	420	35	23.0		
Rise 'N' Shine	1	320	34	18.0		
sausage	1	440	34	28.0		
sausage & egg	1	490	35	31.0		
steak	1	500	46	29.0		
steak & eggs	1	550	47	32.0		
Cheeseburger	1	320	33	14.0		
(also see Hamburgers)						
Chicken breast, grilled sandwich	1	310	34	9.0		
Chicken fillet sandwich	1	370	44	13.0		
Chicken Stix regular	1 order	210	13	9.0		
Crispy Curls	1 order	300	36	16.0		
Fisherman's Fillet sandwich	1	500	49	24.0		
French fries, regular	1 order	230	30	11.0		
Hamburger	1	270	33	10.0		
Big Deluxe	1	500	32	30.0		
Mushroom 'N' Swiss	1	490	33	27.0		
Quarter pound burger w/cheese	1	500	34	29.0		
regular	1	270	33	10.0		

♥ = HEALTHY HEART FOOD   T = TRIGGER FOOD

Item	SERVING	CAL-ORIES	CARBS (g)	TOTAL FAT(g)	♥	T
Hash rounds	1 order	230	24	14.0		
Hot dog	1	300	25	17.0		T
Hot Ham 'N' Cheese	1	330	32	12.0		
Ice cream						
Cool Twist cone, chocolate	1	200	31	6.0		
Cool Twist cone, vanilla	1	190	28	6.0		
Cool Twist sundae, hot fudge	1	320	45	12.0		
Pancakes						
regular	1 order	280	56	2.0	♥	
w/bacon	1 order	350	56	9.0		
w/sausage	1 order	430	56	16.0		
Roast Beef sandwich						
Big Roast Beef	1	300	32	11.0		
regular	1	260	31	9.0		
Salads						
Chef	1	240	5	15.0		T
Chicken 'n' pasta	1	230	23	3.0	♥	T
garden	1	210	3	14.0		
side	1	20	1	0.4	♥	
Shake						
chocolate	1	460	85	8.0		
vanilla	1	400	66	9.0		
Turkey Club sandwich	1	390	32	16.0		
Jack in the Box						
Breakfast Jack	1 order	307	30	13.0		
Cheeseburger						
double	1	467	33	27.0		
regular	1	315	33	14.0		
w/bacon	1	705	48	39.0		
(also see Hamburgers)						
Chicken fajita pita	1	292	29	8.0		
Chicken fillet sandwich, grilled	1	408	33	17.0		
Chicken strips, 4 pieces	1 order	349	28	14.0		
Chicken sandwich, supreme	1	575	34	36.0		
Crescent Canadian	1 serv.	452	25	31.0		
Crescent Supreme	1 serv.	547	27	40.0		
Egg rolls, 3 pieces	1 order	405	42	19.0		
Eggs, see Scrambled egg platter						
Fish sandwich, supreme	1	554	47	32.0		
French fries, regular	1 order	353	43	19.0		
Hamburgers						
Jumbo Jack	1	584	42	34.0		

♥ = HEALTHY HEART FOOD   T = TRIGGER FOOD

Item	SERVING	CAL-ORIES	CARBS (g)	TOTAL FAT(g)	♥	T
Jumbo Jack w/cheese	1	667	46	40.0		
regular	1	267	28	11.0		
Hash browns	1 order	116	11	7.0		
Onion rings, regular	1 order	382	39	23.0		
Pancake platter	1 order	612	87	22.0		
Salads						
chef	1	295	3	18.0		T
Mexican chicken	1	442	30	23.0		T
side	1	51	1	3.0		
taco	1	503	28	31.0		T
Scrambled egg platter	1	662	52	40.0		
Shake						
chocolate	1	330	55	7.0		
vanilla	1	320	57	6.0		
Shrimp, 10 pieces	1 order	270	22	16.0		
Taquitos, 5 pieces	1 order	363	40	16.0		
Kentucky Fried Chicken (KFC)						
Chicken						
Extra Crispy						
breast	1 piece	353	14	20.9		
drumstick	1 piece	173	6	10.9		
thigh	1 piece	371	14	26.3		
wing	1 piece	218	8	15.6		
Original recipe						
breast	1 piece	283	9	15.3		
drumstick	1 piece	146	4	8.5		
thigh	1 piece	294	11	19.7		
wing	1 piece	178	6	11.7		
Chicken Little's, sandwiches	1	169	14	10.1		
Chicken sandwich, Colonel's	1	482	39	27.3		
Corn-on-the-cob	1	176	32	3.1	♥	
French fries	1 order	244	31	11.9		
Hot wings	1 order	376	13	24.1		
Kentucky Nuggets	1 piece	46	2	2.9		
Kentucky Nugget sauces						
Barbeque	1 oz.	35	7	0.6	♥	T
Honey	1 oz.	98	24	0.1	♥	T
Mustard	1 oz.	36	6	0.9		T
Sweet & sour	1 oz.	58	13	0.6	♥	T
Mashed potatoes & gravy	1 order	71	12	1.6		
McDonald's						
Apple pie	1 serv.	260	30	14.8		

♥ = HEALTHY HEART FOOD   T = TRIGGER FOOD

Item	SERVING	CAL-ORIES	CARBS (g)	TOTAL FAT(g)	♥	T
Biscuit						
w/bacon, egg, & cheese	1	440	33	26.4		
w/biscuit spread	1	260	32	12.7		
w/sausage	1	440	32	29.0		
w/sausage & egg	1	520	33	34.5		
Cheeseburger	1	310	31	13.8		
(also see Hamburgers)						
Chicken McNuggets	1 serv.	290	17	16.3		
Chicken sandwich, McChicken	1	490	40	28.6		
Cookies, McDonaldland	1 serv.	290	47	9.2		
Danish, apple	1	390	51	17.9		
Egg McMuffin	1 serv.	290	28	11.2		
Eggs, see Scrambled eggs						
Filet-O-Fish sandwich	1	440	38	26.1		
French fries, medium	1	320	36	17.1		
Hamburgers						
Big Mac	1	560	43	32.4		
hamburger	1	260	31	9.5		
McDLT	1	580	36	36.8		
McLean Deluxe	1	320	35	10.0		
McLean Deluxe w/cheese	1	370	35	14.0		
Quarter Pounder	1	410	34	20.7		
Quarter Pounder w/cheese	1	520	35	29.2		
Hot cakes w/butter & syrup	1 order	410	74	9.2		
McChicken	1	490	40	28.6		
McMuffins						
sausage	1	370	27	21.9		
sausage w/egg	1	440	28	26.8		
Salads						
Chef	1	230	8	13.3		T
Chunky chicken	1	140	5	3.4		T
garden	1	110	6	6.6		T
side	1	60	3	3.3		
Scrambled eggs	1 order	140	1	9.8		
Shakes						
chocolate	1	320	66	1.7	♥	
vanilla	1	290	60	1.3	♥	
Yogurt						
cone, vanilla	1	100	22	0.8	♥	T
sundae, hot fudge	1	240	51	3.2	♥	
Pizza Hut						
Pizza						
Hand-tossed, medium						

♥ = HEALTHY HEART FOOD   T = TRIGGER FOOD

Item	SERVING	CAL- ORIES	CARBS (g)	TOTAL FAT(g)	♥	T
cheese	1 slice	259	28	10.0		
pepperoni	1 slice	250	25	11.5		
Supreme	1 slice	270	25	13.0		
Super Supreme	1 slice	232	22	10.5		
Pan Pizza, medium						
cheese	1 slice	246	29	9.0		
pepperoni	1 slice	270	31	11.0		
Supreme	1 slice	295	27	15.0		
Super Supreme	1 slice	282	27	13.0		
Personal Pan Pizza						
cheese	1 pie	695	78	27.0		
pepperoni	1 pie	675	76	29.0		
Supreme	1 pie	647	76	28.0		
Thin 'n Crispy						
cheese	1 slice	299	19	8.5		
pepperoni	1 slice	207	18	10.0		
Supreme	1 slice	230	21	11.0		
Super Supreme	1 slice	232	22	5.2		
Roy Rogers						
Cheeseburger	1	552	31	33.0		
Chicken, fried						
breast	1 serv.	412	17	24.0		
drumstick	1 serv.	140	6	8.0		
wing	1 serv.	192	9	13.0		
Crescent sandwich						
regular	1	408	28	27.0		
w/bacon	1	446	28	30.0		
w/sausage	1	464	28	42.0		
Egg & biscuit platter						
regular	1 serv.	557	44	34.0		
w/bacon	1 serv.	607	44	39.0		
w/sausage	1 serv.	713	44	49.0		
Fish sandwich	1	514	58	24.0		
French fries, regular	1 serv.	320	39	16.0		
Hamburgers						
Expressburger	1	561	42	32.0		
regular	1	472	37	25.0		
Pancake platter						
w/syrup & butter	1 serv.	386	63	13.0		
w/syrup, butter, & bacon	1 serv.	436	63	17.0		
w/syrup, butter, & sausage	1 serv.	542	63	28.0		
Roast beef, sandwich						
regular	1	350	37	11.0		

♥ = HEALTHY HEART FOOD   T = TRIGGER FOOD

Item	SERVING	CAL-ORIES	CARBS (g)	TOTAL FAT(g)	♥	T
regular w/cheese	1	403	37	15.0		
Shakes						
chocolate	1	358	61	10.0		
vanilla	1	306	45	11.0		
Sundae, hot fudge	1	337	53	13.0		
Taco Bell						
Burritos						
bean	1 order	447	63	14.0		
beef	1 order	493	48	21.0		
chicken	1 order	334	38	12.0		
combination	1 order	407	46	16.0		
Supreme	1 order	503	55	22.0		
Enchirito w/red sauce	1 order	382	31	20.0		
Meximelt	1 order	266	19	15.0		
Nachos	1 order	346	37	18.0		
Nachos Supreme	1 order	367	41	27.0		
Pintos & cheese w/red sauce	1 order	190	19	9.0		
Taco						
chicken	1	171	11	9.0		
chicken, soft	1	213	19	10.0		
regular	1	183	11	11.0		
regular, soft	1	225	18	12.0		
Supreme	1	230	12	15.0		
Supreme, soft	1	272	19	16.0		
Tostada						
chicken w/red sauce	1	264	20	15.0		
regular w/red sauce	1	243	27	11.0		
Wendy's						
Chicken sandwich, club	1	506	43	25.0		
Chicken sandwich, grilled	1	340	37	13.0		
Chicken	1 order	440	43	19.0		
Chicken nuggets, crispy	6 nuggets	280	12	20.0		
Fish fillet	1	460	42	25.0		
Hamburgers						
Big Classic	1	570	47	33.0		
regular	1	340	30	15.0		
w/everything	1	420	35	21.0		
Salads						
Chef	1	130	8	5.0		T
garden	1	70	9	2.0		T
taco	1	530	55	23.0		T
(see also SuperBar)						

♥ = HEALTHY HEART FOOD   T = TRIGGER FOOD

Item	SERVING	CAL-ORIES	CARBS (g)	TOTAL FAT(g)	♥	T
SuperBar						
cheese sauce	1 serv.	39	5	2.0		T
fettuccini, cheese	1 serv.	190	27	3.0	♥	
medley	1 serv.	60	9	2.0		T
ravioli, cheese	1 serv.	45	8	1.0		
refried beans	1 serv.	70	10	3.0		
rice, Spanish	1 serv.	70	13	1.0	♥	
rotini	1 serv.	90	15	2.0		
taco chips	1 serv.	260	40	10.0		
taco shells	1 serv.	45	6	3.0		
tortellini, cheese	1 serv.	60	12	1.0	♥	
tortilla shell	1 serv.	110	19	3.0		
Potatoes						
baked, plain	1	270	63	0.4	♥	T
french fried	1 order	240	33	12.0		
stuffed w/bacon & cheese	1	520	70	18.0		
stuffed w/broccoli & cheese	1	400	58	16.0		
stuffed w/cheese	1	420	66	15.0		
stuffed w/chili & cheese	1	500	71	18.0		

FATS AND OILS

Item	SERVING	CAL-ORIES	CARBS (g)	TOTAL FAT(g)	♥	T
Butter						
from stick	1 Tbsp.	100	0	11.0		
whipped	1 Tbsp.	80	0	9.0		
Butter substitute						
sesame butter						
paste	1 Tbsp.	85	5	7.3		T
tahini, from toasted kernel	1 Tbsp.	89	3	8.1		T
tahini, from roasted kernels (also see Margarine)	1 Tbsp.	89	3	8.1		T
Lard	1 Tbsp.	115	0	13.0		
Margarine						
imitation	1 Tbsp.	50	0	5.0		
regular, hard	1 Tbsp.	100	0	11.0		
regular, soft	1 Tbsp.	100	0	11.0		
spread, hard	1 Tbsp.	75	0	9.0		

♥ = HEALTHY HEART FOOD   T = TRIGGER FOOD

Item	SERVING	CAL-ORIES	CARBS (g)	TOTAL FAT(g)	♥	T
spread, soft	1 Tbsp.	75	0	9.0		
Mayonnaise	1 Tbsp.	100	0	11.0		
Mayonnaise, substitute						
Hain Eggless	1 Tbsp.	110	0	12.0		
soybean	1 Tbsp.	35	2	2.9		
sunflower	1 Tbsp.	71	1	8.0		
tofu	1 Tbsp.	40	1	4.0		
Oil						
canola	1 Tbsp.	124	0	14.0		
corn	1 Tbsp.	125	0	14.0		
olive	1 Tbsp.	125	0	14.0		
peanut	1 Tbsp.	125	0	14.0		
safflower	1 Tbsp.	125	0	14.0		
soybean-cottonseed blend	1 Tbsp.	125	0	14.0		
soybean, hardened	1 Tbsp.	125	0	14.0		
sunflower	1 Tbsp.	12	0	14.0		
vegetable oil	1 Tbsp.	120	0	14.0		
Shortening, see Vegetable shortening						
Tartar sauce						
Hellman's/Best Foods	1 Tbsp.	70	0	8.0		
most brands	1 Tbsp.	75	1	8.0		T
Vegetable shortening	1 Tbsp.	115	0	13.0		
Vinegar and oil	1 Tbsp.	75	0	8.0		

FRUITS AND JUICES

Item	SERVING	CAL-ORIES	CARBS (g)	TOTAL FAT(g)	♥	T
Apple, dried						
sweetened	1 cup	232	58	0.2	♥	T
unsweetened	1 cup	142	39	0.2	♥	T
Apple, fresh	1 medium	80	21	0.0	♥	T
Apple, fresh	1 large	125	32	1.0	♥	T
Apple juice	8 fl. oz.	115	29	0.0	♥	T
Apple-cranberry juice	8 fl. oz.	124	32	0.0	♥	
Apple-grape juice	8 fl. oz.	117	31	0.0	♥	
Apple-raspberry juice	8 fl. oz.	126	32	0.0	♥	
Applesauce						
sweetened	1 cup	195	51	0.0	♥	
unsweetened	1 cup	125	28	0.0	♥	

♥ = HEALTHY HEART FOOD   T = TRIGGER FOOD

Item	SERVING	CAL-ORIES	CARBS (g)	TOTAL FAT(g)	♥	T
Apricot, canned						
in extra light syrup	1 cup	112	28	0.2	♥	
in heavy syrup	1 cup	215	55	0.0	♥	
in light syrup	1 cup	142	38	0.2	♥	
in water, peeled	1 cup	50	12	1.4		
in water, unpeeled	1 cup	62	13	0.4	♥	
juice pack	1 cup	120	31	0.0	♥	
Apricot, cooked, unsweet-ened	1 cup	215	55	0.0	♥	
Apricot dried						
sweetened	1 cup	232	58	0.4	♥	T
unsweetened	1 cup	142	39	0.4	♥	T
Apricot, fresh	3 apricots	50	12	0.0	♥	
Apricot nectar	1 cup	140	36	0.0	♥	
Avocado						
California	1	305	12	30.0		
Florida	1	340	27	27.0		
Banana	1	105	27	1.0	♥	T
Banana chips, freeze-dried	1 cup	496	30	16.0		T
Blackberries						
canned						
in heavy syrup	1 cup	236	59	0.4	♥	
in water	1 cup	50	8	1.0	♥	
fresh	1 cup	75	18	1.0	♥	
frozen, unsweetened	1 cup	98	24	0.6	♥	
Blueberries						
canned						
in heavy syrup	1 cup	224	56	0.8	♥	
in water	1 cup	80	18	0.0	♥	
fresh	1 cup	80	20.0	1.0	♥	
frozen						
sweetened	1 cup	188	50	0.4	♥	
unsweetened	1 cup	78	19	1.0	♥	
Cantaloupe, medium	½	95	22	1.0	♥	
Carrot juice	8 fl. oz.	97	23	0.4	♥	T
Cherries, sour						
canned						
in extra heavy syrup	1 cup	296	76	0.2	♥	
in heavy syrup	1 cup	232	60	0.2	♥	
in light syrup	1 cup	188	49	0.2	♥	
in water	1 cup	96	22	0.2	♥	
fresh	1 cup	78	19	0.4		
frozen						
unsweetened	1 cup	72	17	0.6	♥	

♥ = HEALTHY HEART FOOD   T = TRIGGER FOOD

Item	SERVING	CAL-ORIES	CARBS (g)	TOTAL FAT(g)	♥	T
Cherries, sweet						
canned						
in extra heavy syrup	1 cup	266	68	0.4	♥	
in heavy syrup	1 cup	214	55	0.4	♥	
in light syrup	1 cup	170	44	0.4	♥	
in water	1 cup	114	29	0.4	♥	
fresh	1 cup	104	24	1.4	♥	
frozen						
sweetened	1 cup	232	58	0.4	♥	
Cranberry juice						
Smucker's Naturally 100%	8 fl. oz.	130	30	0.0	♥	T
sweetened	8 fl. oz.	145	38	0.0	♥	T
Cranberry juice cocktail	8 fl. oz.	140	35	0.0	♥	T
Cranberry sauce	1 cup	420	108	0.0	♥	
Dates	10	230	61	0.0	♥	T
Figs						
canned						
in extra heavy syrup	1 cup	280	73	0.2	♥	
in heavy syrup	1 cup	228	60	0.2	♥	
in light syrup	1 cup	174	45	0.2	♥	
in water	1 cup	130	35	0.2	♥	
dried	10	475	122	2.0	♥	T
Fruit cocktail, canned						
in extra heavy syrup	1 cup	230	60	0.2	♥	
in extra light syrup	1 cup	110	29	0.2	♥	
in heavy syrup	1 cup	186	48	0.2	♥	
juice pack	1 cup	115	29	0.0	♥	T
in light syrup	1 cup	144	38	0.2	♥	
in water	1 cup	80	21	0.2	♥	T
Fruit salad, canned						
in extra heavy syrup	1 cup	228	59	0.2	♥	
in heavy syrup	1 cup	188	49	0.2	♥	
in juice	1 cup	124	32	1.0	♥	T
in light syrup	1 cup	146	38	0.2	♥	
in water	1 cup	74	19	0.2	♥	T
Fruit, mixed						
in heavy syrup	1 cup	184	48	0.2	♥	
in juice, Libby Lite	1 cup	100	28	0.0	♥	T
in light syrup	1 cup	150	40	1.8	♥	
Grapefruit						
canned w/syrup	1 cup	150	39	0.0	♥	
fresh	½	40	10	0.0	♥	T
Grapefruit juice						
sweetened	1 cup	115	28	0.0	♥	

♥ = HEALTHY HEART FOOD   T = TRIGGER FOOD

Item	SERVING	CAL-ORIES	CARBS (g)	TOTAL FAT(g)	♥	T
unsweetened	1 cup	95	22	0.0	♥	T
Grape juice	8 fl. oz.	120	36	0.0	♥	
Kraft, unsweetened	8 fl. oz.	139	33	0.0	♥	
Veryfine 100%	8 fl. oz.	153	37	0.0	♥	
Grapes						
Thompson, seedless	10	35	9	0.0	♥	
Tokay & Emperor, seedless	10	40	10	0.0	♥	
Honeydew	¹⁄₁₀	45	12	0.0	♥	
Kiwifruit	1	45	11	0.0	♥	
Lemon	1	15	5	0.0	♥	
Lemon juice	1 Tbsp.	5	1	0.0	♥	
Limeade, canned	8 fl. oz.	94	25	0.0	♥	
Mango	1	135	35	1.0	♥	
Nectarine	1	65	16	1.0	♥	
Orange	1 medium	60	15	0.0	♥	T
Orange drink, Hi-C	8 fl. oz.	127	31	0.6	♥	
Orange-grapefruit juice	8 fl. oz.	105	25	0.0	♥	
Orange juice	8 fl. oz.	110	26	0.0	♥	T
Orange juice drink, Tropicana sparkler	8 fl. oz.	110	26	0.0	♥	
Papaya	8 fl. oz.	65	17	0.0	♥	
Peach						
canned						
heavy syrup	1 cup	190	51	0.0	♥	
juice pack	1 cup	110	29	0.0	♥	T
dried	1 cup	380	98	1.0	♥	T
fresh	1	35	10	0.0	♥	T
Pear						
canned						
heavy syrup	1 cup	190	49	0.0	♥	
juice pack	1 cup	125	32	0.0	♥	T
fresh	1	100	21	1.0	♥	T
Pineapple						
canned						
in heavy syrup,	1 slice	90	23.0	0.0	♥	
in juice pack	1 slice	70	17.5	0.5	♥	T
fresh	1 slice	39	11.0	0.0	♥	T
Pineapple juice, unsweetened	8 fl. oz.	140	34	0.0	♥	T
Plantains						
cooked	1 cup	180	48	0.0	♥	
fresh	1 cup	184	50	1.0	♥	
Plum						
canned						
in heavy syrup	1 cup	230	60	0.0	♥	

♥ = HEALTHY HEART FOOD   T = TRIGGER FOOD

Item	SERVING	CAL-ORIES	CARBS (g)	TOTAL FAT(g)	♥	T
juice pack	1 cup	145	38	0.0	♥	T
fresh						
large	1	35	9	0.0	♥	T
small	1	15	4	0.0	♥	T
Prune juice	8 fl. oz.	180	45	0.0	♥	T
Prunes, dried						
cooked, unsweetened	1 cup	225	60	0.0	♥	T
uncooked	4–5	115	31	0.0	♥	T
Raisins, seedless	2 oz.	160	44	0.0	♥	T
Raspberries						
fresh	1 cup	60	14	1.0	♥	
frozen, sweetened	1 cup	255	65	0.0	♥	
Rhubarb, cooked, sweetened	1 cup	280	75	0.0	♥	
Strawberries						
fresh	1 cup	45	10	1.0		T
frozen, sweetened	1 cup	245	66	0.0	♥	
Tangerine						
canned, light syrup	1 cup	155	41	0.0	♥	
fresh	1	35	9	0.0	♥	T
Tangerine juice, sweetened	8 fl. oz.	125	30	0.0	♥	
Tomato juice,						
canned	8 fl. oz.	40	10	0.0	♥	T
Hunt's, canned	8 fl. oz.	40	9	0.0	♥	T
Hunt's, canned, no salt added	8 fl. oz.	60	15	0.0	♥	T
Vegetable juice cocktail	8 fl. oz.	45	11	0.0	♥	T
Vegetable juice, V-8	8 fl. oz.	47	11	0.0	♥	T
Watermelon	4" × 8" wedge	155	35	2.0	♥	T

GRAVIES AND SAUCES

Item	SERVING	CAL-ORIES	CARBS (g)	TOTAL FAT(g)	♥	T
Au jus gravy						
French's mix	¼ cup	10	2	0.0	♥	
Heinz HomeStyle, canned	¼ cup	18	2	1.0		
Barbecue sauce						
bottled	1 Tbsp.	10	2	0.0	♥	T
Heinz Old Fashioned	1 Tbsp.	18	4	0.1	♥	T
Kraft Thick'n Spicy Original	1 Tbsp.	25	6	0.5	♥	T

♥ = HEALTHY HEART FOOD   T = TRIGGER FOOD

Item	SERVING	CAL-ORIES	CARBS (g)	TOTAL FAT(g)	♥	T
Beef gravy						
canned	¼ cup	30	3	1.0		
Franco American, canned	¼ cup	25	4	1.0		
Brown gravy						
French's mix	¼ cup	20	4	1.0		
Heinz HomeStyle, canned	¼ cup	25	3	1.0		
Cheese sauce, w/milk	¼ cup	77	6	4.3		
Chicken gravy						
canned	¼ cup	48	3	3.5		
French's mix	¼ cup	25	4	1.0		
from mix	¼ cup	21	4	0.5		
Heinz HomeStyle, canned	¼ cup	35	3	2.0		
Chili sauce, Heinz	1 Tbsp.	16	4	0.0	♥	T
Clam sauce						
Progresso Authentic, refrig.	¼ cup	65	2	4.5		
red, Progresso, canned	¼ cup	35	4	1.5		
white, Progresso, canned	¼ cup	55	1	4.0		
Cocktail sauce	1 Tbsp.	15	4	0.1	♥	T
Cranberry sauce w/other fruit	¼ cup	100	24	0.0	♥	
Hollandaise sauce	¼ cup	384	0	42.0		
Mushroom gravy						
canned	¼ cup	30	3	1.5		
French's mix	¼ cup	20	3	1.0		
Heinz HomeStyle, canned	¼ cup	25	3	1.0		
Onion gravy						
French's mix	¼ cup	25	4	1.0		T
Pasta sauce						
Marinara	¼ cup	45	5	2.5		
meat	¼ cup	55	7	2.5		
mushroom	¼ cup	55	7	2.5		
pesto	¼ cup	40	2	2.0		
primavera	¼ cup	95	4	8.5		
Picante sauce, all varieties	¼ cup	16	4	0.4		
Pizza sauce						
plain	¼ cup	30	5	1.0		T
w/pepperoni	¼ cup	40	5	2.0		T
Pork gravy						
French's mix	¼ cup	20	4	1.0		
Heinz HomeStyle, canned	¼ cup	25	3	1.0		
Salsa sauce, Old El Paso Thick'n Chunky	¼ cup	12	2	0.0	♥	
Sour cream sauce, mix	¼ cup	128	12	7.6		
Soy sauce						
bottled	1 Tbsp.	10	2	0.0	♥	T

♥ = HEALTHY HEART FOOD   T = TRIGGER FOOD

Item	SERVING	CAL-ORIES	CARBS (g)	TOTAL FAT(g)	♥	T
from soy & wheat (shoyu)	1 Tbsp.	9	2	0.0	♥	T
from soy (tamari)	1 Tbsp.	11	1	0.6		T
Kikkoman	1 Tbsp.	10	1	0.0	♥	T
Steak sauce						
A-1	1 Tbsp.	12	3	0.0	♥	
French's	1 Tbsp.	25	6	0.0	♥	
Stroganoff sauce	¼ cup	68	9	2.7		
Tartar sauce						
Great Impressions	1 Tbsp.	86	1	9.0		
Heinz	1 Tbsp.	71	2	7.2		
Teriyaki sauce						
Kikkoman	1 Tbsp.	15	3	0.0	♥	T
Turkey gravy						
Heinz HomeStyle, canned	¼ cup	25	3	1.0		
Lawry's mix	¼ cup	26	3	1.0		
White sauce						
from mix	¼ cup	60	5	3.3		
homemade	¼ cup	98	6	5.0		
Worcestershire sauce, Lea & Perrins	1 Tbsp.	5	1	0.7		

MEATS

Item	SERVING	CAL-ORIES	CARBS (g)	TOTAL FAT(g)	♥	T

Note: All values are for meats broiled, braised, or roasted unless otherwise noted. For lunch meats, hot dogs, and sausages, see our Processed Meats section.

Item	SERVING	CAL-ORIES	CARBS (g)	TOTAL FAT(g)	♥	T
Beef						
bottom round						
lean	3 oz.	186	0	9.0		
regular	3 oz.	220	0	13.0		
brisket						
lean	3 oz.	206	0	10.9		
regular	3 oz.	328	0	26.9		
chuck, arm, pot roast						
lean	3 oz.	191	0	7.9		
regular	3 oz.	296	0	21.9		
chuck, blade roast						
lean	3 oz.	232	0	12.0		

Item	SERVING	CAL-ORIES	CARBS (g)	TOTAL FAT(g)	♥	T
regular	3 oz.	325	0	26.0		
corned beef	3 oz.	214	1	16.1		
eye of round						
lean	3 oz.	148	0	4.9		
regular	3 oz.	205	0	12.0		
flank steak, lean	3 oz.	224	0	13.9		
full out round,						
lean	3 oz.	163	0	6.2		
regular	3 oz.	204	0	11.6		
ground beef						
extra lean	3 oz.	218	0	13.9		
lean	3 oz.	231	0	15.7		
regular	3 oz.	246	0	17.6		
rib, large end						
lean	3 oz.	213	0	12.5		
regular	3 oz.	250	0	27.1		
rib, small end						
lean	3 oz.	197	0	11.1		
regular	3 oz.	282	0	23.5		
rib, whole						
lean	3 oz.	207	0	11.9		
regular	3 oz.	320	0	26.5		
roast						
lean	3 oz.	205	0	12.0		
regular	3 oz.	315	0	26.0		
shank, cross out						
lean	3 oz.	171	0	5.4		
regular	3 oz.	224	0	12.4		
short ribs						
lean	3 oz.	251	0	15.4		
regular	3 oz.	400	0	35.7		
steak, Porterhouse						
lean	3 oz.	185	0	9.1		
regular	3 oz.	260	0	18.8		
steak, sirloin						
lean	3 oz.	180	0	7.0		
regular	3 oz.	240	0	15.0		
steak, T-bone						
lean	3 oz.	182	0	8.9		
regular	3 oz.	254	0	18.0		
tenderloin						
lean	3 oz.	189	0	9.5		
regular	3 oz.	259	0	18.6		

♥ = HEALTHY HEART FOOD   T = TRIGGER FOOD

Item	SERVING	CAL-ORIES	CARBS (g)	TOTAL FAT(g)	♥	T
tip round						
lean	3 oz.	160	0	6.2		
regular	3 oz.	210	0	12.7		
top loin						
lean	3 oz.	182	0	8.6		
regular	3 oz.	254	0	17.9		
top round						
lean, broiled	3 oz.	160	0	5.0		
lean, fried	3 oz.	193	0	7.3		
regular, broiled	3 oz.	190	0	9.0		
regular, fried	3 oz.	236	0	13.1		
top sirloin						
lean, broiled	3 oz.	172	0	6.8		
lean, fried	3 oz.	202	0	9.3		
regular, broiled	3 oz.	229	0	14.2		
regular, fried	3 oz.	278	0	19.4		
Beefalo	3 oz.	165	0	5.3		
Brains						
beef, fried	3 oz.	166	0	13.5		
lamb, fried	3 oz.	232	0	18.9		
pork, braised	3 oz.	117	0	8.1		
Heart						
beef	3 oz.	149	1	4.8		
chicken	3 oz.	158	0	6.8		
lamb	3 oz.	158	2	6.8		
pork	3 oz.	126	1	4.3		
turkey	3 oz.	151	2	5.2		
Kidney						
beef	3 oz.	122	1	2.9		
lamb	3 oz.	116	1	3.1		
pork	3 oz.	128	0	4.0		
Lamb						
chops, arm						
lean	3 oz.	238	0	12.0		
regular	3 oz.	300	0	20.0		
chops, loin						
lean	3 oz.	183	0	8.0		
regular	3 oz.	252	0	17.0		
leg						
lean	3 oz.	162	0	7.0		
regular	3 oz.	205	0	13.0		
rib						
lean	3 oz.	200	0	11.0		
regular	3 oz.	307	0	25.2		

♥ = HEALTHY HEART FOOD   T = TRIGGER FOOD

Item	SERVING	CAL-ORIES	CARBS (g)	TOTAL FAT(g)	♥	T
Liver						
beef, pan-fried	3 oz.	184	7	6.8		
chicken, simmered	3 oz.	134	1	4.7		
pork, braised	3 oz.	140	3	3.8		
turkey, simmered	3 oz.	144	3	5.0		
Pancreas						
beef	3 oz.	230	0	14.6		
lamb	3 oz.	199	0	12.8		
pork	3 oz.	186	0	9.1		
Pork						
bacon						
Canadian, cooked	3 oz.	105	0	4.2		
cooked	3 slices	120	0	9.3		
raw	3 slices	468	0	48.0		
chop, loin						
lean, broiled	3 oz.	190	0	10.0		
lean, pan-fried	3 oz.	225	0	14.0		
regular, broiled	3 oz.	266	0	18.0		
regular, pan-fried	3 oz.	324	0	11.0		
ham, cured						
lean	3 oz.	131	0	5.0		
regular	3 oz.	205	0	14.0		
ham (leg)						
lean	3 oz.	192	0	10.0		
regular	3 oz.	250	0	18.0		
rib roast						
lean	3 oz.	210	0	12.0		
regular	3 oz.	270	0	20.0		
shoulder						
lean	3 oz.	206	0	10.0		
regular	3 oz.	295	0	22.0		
Rabbit						
roasted	3 oz.	131	0	5.4		
stewed	3 oz.	176	0	7.1		
Tongue						
beef	3 oz.	241	0	17.6		
lamb	3 oz.	234	0	17.2		
pork	3 oz.	230	0	15.8		
Veal						
cutlet						
braised or broiled	3 oz.	185	0	9.0		
breaded, fried	3 oz.	220	17	12.0		
roasted	3 oz.	230	0	14.0		

♥ = HEALTHY HEART FOOD   T = TRIGGER FOOD

Item	SERVING	CAL-ORIES	CARBS (g)	TOTAL FAT(g)	♥	T
leg of veal						
lean	3 oz.	128	0	2.8		
regular	3 oz.	136	0	4.0		
loin						
lean	3 oz.	148	0	5.9		
regular	3 oz.	184	0	10.5		
rib						
lean	3 oz.	151	0	6.3		
regular	3 oz.	194	0	11.9		
shoulder blade						
lean	3 oz.	146	0	5.8		
regular	3 oz.	158	0	7.3		
sirloin						
lean	3 oz.	143	0	5.3		
regular	3 oz.	172	0	8.9		
Venison	3 oz.	134	0	2.7	♥	

Medications, vitamins, and supplements, particularly cough syrups, drops, and lozenges can be very high in carbohydrates. Taken at times other than at your Reward Meal, they may trigger carbohydrate hunger, cravings, and weight gain for the carbohydrate addict.

The carbohydrate counts listed here are for "available" carbohydrates, that is, those that may be absorbed by your body. In addition, nonavailable carbohydrates in these medications and supplements may also increase carbohydrate cravings and weight gain. These carbohydrate counts are usually not listed. Stool softeners, in particular, may be high in nonavailable carbohydrates.

Trigger designations (T) indicated those medications and supplements that have been found to trigger cravings and weight gain. As always, the importance of the use of medications and supplements must be weighed against difficulties that they might present, and *in all instances, check with your physician.*

Fat levels for these items are usually negligible, therefore no fat counts (and no Healthy Heart designations) have been included in this section.

Item	DOSE	CAL-ORIES	CARBS (g)	T
Capsules & Tablets				
Acetaminophen, 325-mg	1	0	0	T
Acetaminophen, 500-mg	1	0	0	T
Aspirin	1	0	0	T
BQ Cold Tablets	1	0	0	
Bufferin	1	0	0	T
Bufferin, Arthritis Strength	1	0	0	T
Comtrex	1	0	0	
Datril, 5-grain	1	0	0	
Datril, 7.5-grain	1	0	0	
Excedrin	1	0	0	T
Excedrin, PM	1	0	0	
4-Way Cold Tablets	1	1	0	
Gelusil	1	3	1	T
Gelusil II	1	4	1	
Lomotil	1	0	0	
Migral	1	0	0	
Milk of Magnesia	1	1	0	
Mycostatin Oral	1	0	0	

T = TRIGGER FOOD

Item	DOSE	CAL-ORIES	CARBS (g)	T
Rolaids	1	4	1	T
Sine-Aid Tablets	1	0	0	
Sudafed, 30-mg	1	0	0	
Tylenol	1	0	0	T
Tylenol, Extra Strength	1	1	0	T
Cough Drops & Lozenges				
Black, Beech-Nut	1	10	2	
Cherry, Hall's	1	15	4	T
Cough suppressant lozenges	1	16	0	T
Decongestant lozenges	1	16	0	T
Honey, Pine Brothers	1	8	2	T
Lemon, Hall's	1	15	4	T
Listerine Throat Lozenges	1	8	2	
Menthol, Beech-Nut	1	10	2	
Menthol-Lyptus, Hall's	1	15	4	
Spec T Sore Throat Anesthetic	1	16	0	
Wild Cherry, Beech-Nut	1	10	2	T
Wild Cherry, Pine Brothers	1	8	2	T
Cough Syrups & Expectorants				
Actifed	1 tsp.	14	3	T
Comtrex	1 tsp.	14	3	T
CoTylenol	1 tsp.	17	4	T
Extra-Strength Tylenol	1 tsp.	11	3	T
Sudafed	1 tsp.	14	3	T
Triaminic Expectorant	1 tsp.	16	4	T
Triaminic Expectorant DH	1 tsp.	11	3	
Triaminic Syrup	1 tsp.	15	3	T
Vitamins & Mineral Supplements				
Iron w/vitamin C	1	11	0	
Monsters	1	3	1	T
Monsters w/iron	1	2	1	T
Multi-vitamin w/iron	1	1	0	
Pals	1	3	1	T
Pals w/iron	1	2	1	
Rose hips	1	3	1	T
Theragran Tablets	1	1	0	T
Theragran M Tablets	1	0	0	T
Vitamin C	1	3	1	T

T = TRIGGER FOOD

Item	SERVING	CAL-ORIES	CARBS (g)	TOTAL FAT(g)	♥	T
Baking powder	1 tsp.	5	1	0.0	♥	
Catsup	1 Tbsp.	15	4	0.0	♥	T
Celery seed	1 tsp.	10	1	1.0		
Chili powder	1 tsp.	10	1	0.0	♥	T
Chocolate, bitter or baking	1 oz.	145	8	15.0		
Cinnamon	1 tsp.	5	2	0.0	♥	
Cocoa powder w/o dry milk	¾ oz.	75	19	1.0	♥	
Curry powder	1 tsp.	5	1	0.0	♥	
Garlic powder	1 tsp.	10	2	0.0	♥	
Gelatin, dry	1 enve.	25	0	0.0	♥	
Mustard, prepared yellow	1 tsp.	5	0	0.0	♥	T
Olives						
green, medium	3	11	0	1.5		
ripe, medium	3	20	0	2.5		
Onion powder	1 tsp.	5	2	0.0	♥	
Oregano	1 tsp.	5	1	0.0	♥	
Paprika	1 tsp.	5	1	0.0	♥	
Pepper, black	1 tsp.	5	1	0.0	♥	
Pickles						
dill, medium	1	5	1	0.0	♥	
fresh-pack slices	2	10	3	0.0	♥	T
sweet, gherkin	1	20	5	0.0	♥	T
Relish, sweet, chopped	1 Tbsp.	20	5	0.0	♥	T
Salt	1 tsp.	0	0	0.0	♥	
Soy sauce						
bottled	1 Tbsp.	10	2	0.0	♥	T
from soy & wheat (shoyu)	1 Tbsp.	9	2	0.0	♥	T
from soy (tamari)	1 Tbsp.	11	1	0.6		T
Kikkoman	1 Tbsp.	10	1	0.0	♥	T
Tartar sauce						
Great Impressions	1 Tbsp.	86	1	9.0		
Heinz	1 Tbsp.	71	2	7.2		
homemade	1 Tbsp.	75	1	8.0		
Teriyaki sauce						
Kikkoman	1 Tbsp.	15	3	0.0	♥	T
Worcestershire sauce, Lea & Perrins	1 Tbsp.	5	1	0.7		
Vinegar						
basal	1 Tbsp.	7	1	0.0	♥	T
cider	1 Tbsp.	2	1	0.0	♥	
raspberry	1 Tbsp.	7	1	0.0	♥	
red wine	1 Tbsp.	7	1	0.0	♥	T
white, distilled	1 Tbsp.	2	0	0.0	♥	T

♥ = HEALTHY HEART FOOD   T = TRIGGER FOOD

Item	SERVING	CAL-ORIES	CARBS (g)	TOTAL FAT(g)	♥	T
Yeast						
Baker's dry, active	1 pkg.	20	3	0.0	♥	
Brewer's	1 Tbsp.	25	3	0.0	♥	

NUTS, NUT BUTTERS, BEANS, AND SEEDS

Item	SERVING	CAL-ORIES	CARBS (g)	TOTAL FAT(g)	♥	T
Note: All values are for foods that are cooked unless otherwise indicated.						
Adzuki bean, sweetened	1 cup	702	163	0.1	♥	
Adzuki bean, unsweetened	1 cup	646	123	1.0	♥	T
Alfalfa sprouts	1 cup	10	1	0.1	♥	
Almonds	1 oz.	165	6	15.0		
Baked beans						
plain						
S&W Brick Oven	½ cup	160	28	2.0	♥	T
Van Camp's	½ cup	130	26	1.0	♥	
w/franks	½ cup	163	26	7.7		
w/pork	½ cup	130	22	2.0	♥	
Beans						
baked, see Baked beans						
black						
boiled	½ cup	113	20	0.5	♥	
canned, Progresso	½ cup	90	19	1	♥	
broad						
boiled	½ cup	93	17	0.3	♥	
canned	½ cup	91	16	0.3	♥	
Great Northern Bean						
boiled	½ cup	104	19	0.4	♥	
canned	½ cup	80	18	1.0	♥	
green bean						
boiled	½ cup	22	5	0.2	♥	
canned	½ cup	16	4	0.0	♥	
frozen	½ cup	16	4	0.0	♥	
kidney						
boiled, all varieties	½ cup	112	20	0.4	♥	
canned, red	½ cup	100	21	0.8	♥	
canned, red, dark	½ cup	120	22	1.0	♥	
canned, white	½ cup	80	19	0.7	♥	

♥ = HEALTHY HEART FOOD   T = TRIGGER FOOD

Item	SERVING	CAL-ORIES	CARBS (g)	TOTAL FAT(g)	♥	T
lima						
boiled, baby beans	½ cup	115	21	0.3	♥	
boiled, large beans	½ cup	108	20	0.4	♥	
canned	½ cup	100	19	1.0	♥	
frozen	½ cup	100	19	0.0	♥	
mung						
boiled	½ cup	107	19	0.4	♥	
canned	½ cup	8	1	0.6		
pinto						
boiled	½ cup	117	22	0.4	♥	
canned	½ cup	110	21	0.7	♥	
red, Van Camp's	½ cup	97	19	0.3	♥	
refried, canned						
plain	½ cup	130	20	2.0	♥	
w/cheese	½ cup	72	8	2.0		
soy, see Soybeans or individual names of foods in this section						
Black-eyed peas	½ cup	95	18	0.5	♥	
Brazil nuts, shelled	1 oz.	185	4	19.0		
Cashews						
dry roasted	1 oz.	165	9	13.0		T
roasted in oil	1 oz.	165	8	14.0		T
Chestnuts, roasted	1 oz.	68	15	0.3	♥	T
Chick-peas						
boiled	½ cup	134	23	2.1	♥	
canned w/liquid	½ cup	143	27	1.4	♥	T
Coconut						
dried, shredded, sweet	½ cup	235	22	17.0		
fresh, pieces	1 piece	160	7	15.0		T
fresh, shredded	½ cup	143	6	14.0		
Filberts	1 oz.	180	4	18.0		
Garbanzos						
boiled	½ cup	134	22	2.1	♥	
canned w/liquid	½ cup	143	27	1.4	♥	T
Hummus	½ cup	210	25	10.4		
Lentils	½ cup	108	19	0.5	♥	
Lima beans						
cooked	½ cup	130	25	0.5	♥	
frozen/canned	½ cup	140	17	0.5	♥	
Macadamia nuts	1 oz.	205	4	22.0		
Miso, paste	½ cup	235	33	6.5		T
Mixed nuts						
dry roasted	1 oz.	170	7	15.0		T
roasted in oil	1 oz.	175	6	15.0		
Navy, cooked	½ cup	113	20	0.5	♥	

♥ = HEALTHY HEART FOOD   T = TRIGGER FOOD

Item	SERVING	CAL-ORIES	CARBS (g)	TOTAL FAT(g)	♥	T
Peanut butter (2 Tbsps.)	1 oz.	190	6	16.0		T
Peanuts						
dry roasted	1 oz.	164	6	13.9		T
roasted in oil	1 oz.	163	5	13.8		
Pecans, halves	1 oz.	190	5	19.0		
Pine nuts, shelled	1 oz.	160	5	17.0		
Pinto beans	½ cup	133	25	0.5	♥	
Pistachio nuts, shelled	1 oz.	165	7	14.0		
Pumpkin seeds	1 oz.	155	5	13.0		
Sesame seeds	1 Tbsp.	45	1	4.0		
Soybeans						
cooked	½ cup	127	10	5.8		T
miso paste	½ cup	235	33	6.5		T
tempeh	½ cup	165	14	1.4	♥	T
tofu, raw, firm	½ cup	183	5	11.0		
Snap beans, cooked	½ cup	18	5	0.0	♥	
Split peas	½ cup	116	21	0.4	♥	
Squash seeds, dry	1 oz.	155	5	13.0		
Sunflower seeds	1 oz.	160	5	14.0		T
Tahini (2 Tbsps.)	1 oz.	180	6	16.0		T
Tempeh	½ cup	165	14	1.4	♥	T
Tofu, raw	1 square	85	3	5.0		
Walnuts, shelled	1 oz.	175	4	17.0		

POULTRY

Item	SERVING	CAL-ORIES	CARBS (g)	TOTAL FAT(g)	♥	T
Capon, roasted w/skin	3 oz.	195	0	9.9		
Chicken, canned	3 oz.	141	0	7.0		
Chicken hot dog	1	115	3	9.0		T
Chicken						
fried, batter dipped						
breast w/skin	½	365	13	18.0		
drumstick w/skin	1	195	6	11.0		
thigh	1	294	11	19.7		
wing	1	178	6	11.7		
fried, flour coated						
breast w/skin	½	220	2	9.0		
dark meat, no skin	3 oz.	242	4	14.4		
drumstick w/skin	1	120	1	7.0		

♥ = HEALTHY HEART FOOD   T = TRIGGER FOOD

Item	SERVING	CAL-ORIES	CARBS (g)	TOTAL FAT(g)	♥	T
light meat, no skin	3 oz.	209	2	10.3		
mixed meat w/skin	3 oz.	229	3	12.7		
roasted						
breast, no skin	½	140	0	3.0	♥	
dark meat, no skin	3 oz.	174	0	8.2		
drumstick, no skin	1	75	0	2.0		
drumstick w/skin	1	112	0	5.8		
leg (whole) w/skin	1	265	0	15.4		
light, no skin	3 oz.	147	0	3.8		
mixed meat, no skin	3 oz.	161	0	6.3		
mixed meat w/skin	3 oz.	203	0	11.6		
thigh w/skin	1	153	0	9.6		
wing w/skin	1	99	0	6.6		
stewed						
mixed meat, no skin	3 oz.	202	0	10.1		
mixed meat w/skin	3 oz.	242	0	16.0		
Chicken heart	3 oz.	158	0	6.8		
Chicken liver, simmered	3 oz.	134	1	4.7		
Chicken roll, see our Processed Meat section						
Chicken salad (3 oz. scoop)						
commercial	3 oz.	192	9	15.0		T
homemade	3 oz.	190	1	15.0		
Cornish hen w/skin	3 oz.	193	0	10.5		
Duck, roasted						
no skin	3 oz.	171	0	9.5		
w/skin	3 oz.	286	0	24.1		
Goose, roasted						
no skin	3 oz.	202	0	10.8		
w/skin	3 oz.	260	0	18.7		
Pheasant, roasted	3 oz.	185	0	8.1		
Quail, roasted	3 oz.	186	0	8.1		
Squab	3 oz.	120	0	6.3		
Turkey heart	3 oz.	151	2	5.2		
Turkey liver, simmered	3 oz.	144	3	5.0		
Turkey patties, batter/breaded	1	180	10	12.0		
Turkey, roasted						
back meat w/skin	3 oz.	207	0	12.2		
breast w/skin	3 oz.	160	0	6.3		
dark meat, no skin	3 oz.	159	0	6.2		
dark meat w/skin	3 oz.	188	0	9.8		
leg w/skin	3 oz.	177	0	8.3		
light meat, no skin	3 oz.	134	0	2.8	♥	
light meat w/skin	3 oz.	167	0	7.1		
mixed meat, no skin	3 oz.	145	0	4.2		

♥ = HEALTHY HEART FOOD   T = TRIGGER FOOD

Item	SERVING	CAL-ORIES	CARBS (g)	TOTAL FAT(g)	♥	T
mixed meat w/skin, mixed	3 oz.	177	0	8.2		
wing w/skin	3 oz.	195	0	10.6		
Turkey lunch meat, also see our Processed Meat section						

PROCESSED MEATS

Item	SERVING	CAL-ORIES	CARBS (g)	TOTAL FAT(g)	♥	T
Bacon	1 slice	33	0	3.1		T
Bacon, thick-sliced	1 slice	64	0	5.7		T
Bacon, beef	1 slice	50	1	3.5		
Bacon, Canadian	1 slice	35	0	1.4		
Bacon substitute						
beef, Sizzlelean	1 slice	35	0	2.5		
pork, Sizzlelean	1 slice	45	0	4.0		
Beef jerky, Slim Jim Super	1 piece	30	1	1.0		T
Beef loaf	1 oz.	87	1	7.4		
Bologna						
all beef	1 oz.	90	1	3.0		T
beef & pork	1 oz.	80	1	7.0		T
Bratwurst	1 link	310	1	30.0		T
Braunschweiger	1 oz.	80	0	7.0		
Chicken, sliced	1 oz.	60	1	5.0		
Chicken breast, sliced						
most brands	1 oz.	30	1	0.8		
smoked, Deli Select	1 oz.	31	1	0.2	♥	
Chicken ham, sliced	1 oz.	35	1	1.8		T
Chicken roll	1 oz.	35	0	1.2		T
Corned beef	1 oz.	71	0	5.4		
Corned beef hash, Dinty Moore	1 oz.	65	0	4.0		T
Corned beef, lite	1 oz.	35	1	1.0		
Frankfurter	1	180	2	16.0		T
Ham						
baked						
honey lite/lean	1 oz.	31	1	0.8		T
lite/lean	1 oz.	31	1	0.9		T
lite/lean low salt	1 oz.	20	1	0.7		T
most brands	1 oz.	50	0	1.1		T
boiled, Oscar Mayer	1 oz.	33	1	1.0		
canned, spiced	1 oz.	93	1	8.7		

♥ = HEALTHY HEART FOOD   T = TRIGGER FOOD

Item	SERVING	CAL-ORIES	CARBS (g)	TOTAL FAT(g)	♥	T
chopped	1 oz.	41	1	2.3		T
smoked	1 oz.	40	1	2.0		
Hot dog	1	180	2	16.0		T
Kielbasa (Polish sausage)						
lite/lean	1 oz.	72	1	6.0		
most brands	1 oz.	95	1	8.5		T
Knockwurst						
Hebrew National	1 link	263	1	25.0		T
most brands	1 link	180	1	16.0		
Olive loaf	1 oz.	60	1	4.5		
Pastrami	1 oz.	40	1	1.5		
Pickle loaf	1 oz.	80	2	6.0		
Pimento loaf	1 oz.	66	4	1.5		
Porkloaf	1 oz.	80	2	6.3		
Pork & beef	1 oz.	100	1	9.1		
Roast beef						
lite/lean	1 oz.	35	1	1.0		
most brands	1 oz.	40	1	1.0		
Salami						
beef						
Hebrew National	1 oz.	80	1	7.0		T
most brands	1 oz.	60	1	4.0		
cotto						
regular	1 oz.	70	1	6.0		T
turkey	1 oz.	50	1	4.0		
dry/hard	1 oz.	120	0	10.0		T
Genoa	1 oz.	110	0	10.0		T
Sausage						
Brown & serve type	1	70	0	6.5		T
Brown & serve type, lean	1	60	1	5.0		T
Italian, hot	1	180	1	17.0		
Italian, sweet/mild	1	190	1	17.0		
Turkey breast						
glazed	1 oz.	30	1	1.0		T
lean, lite w/skin	1 oz.	35	0	1.0		T
lean, lite w/o skin	1 oz.	26	1	0.2	♥	T
sliced, most brands	1 oz.	30	1	1.0		T
smoked	1 oz.	35	1	1.0		
Turkey bologna	1 oz.	70	2	6.0		T
Turkey pastrami	1 oz.	30	0	1.0		
Turkey roll, white meat	1 oz.	29	1	0.9		T
Turkey salami	1 oz.	50	1	4.0		T
Turkey salami, cotto	1 oz.	50	1	4.0		
Turkey sausage, breakfast	1 oz.	55	1	4.0		T

♥ = HEALTHY HEART FOOD　　　　　　　　　　　　T = TRIGGER FOOD

Item	SERVING	CAL-ORIES	CARBS (g)	TOTAL FAT(g)	♥	T
Turkey sausage, smoked	1 oz.	50	1	3.0		
Vienna sausage	1 oz.	80	1	7.5		T

RICE, PASTA, WHOLE GRAINS, AND NOODLES

Item	SERVING	CAL-ORIES	CARBS (g)	TOTAL FAT(g)	♥	T
Barley	½ cup	88	22	.3	♥	
Buckwheat groats, roasted	½ cup	91	20	0.6	♥	
Bulgur, cooked	½ cup	76	17	0.2	♥	
Corn grits						
instant	1 pkt.	80	18	0.0	♥	
quick	½ cup	73	16	0.0	♥	
regular	½ cup	73	16	0.0	♥	
Cornmeal	½ cup	221	47	2.2	♥	
Couscous						
from grain	½ cup	100	20	0.0	♥	T
pilaf, from mix	½ cup	122	22	3.0		
Hominy grits						
instant	1 pkt.	80	18	0.0	♥	
quick	½ cup	73	16	0.0	♥	
regular	½ cup	73	16	0.0	♥	
Macaroni						
cooked firm	½ cup	85	20	0.5	♥	
cooked tender	½ cup	78	16	0.5	♥	
elbows, whole wheat	½ cup	87	19	0.4	♥	
shells						
protein fortified	½ cup	100	19	0.2	♥	
regular	½ cup	81	17	0.4	♥	
Noodles						
Chinese chow mein	½ cup	119	13	6.9		
egg	½ cup	100	19	1.0	♥	T
Japanese soba, cooked	½ cup	57	12	0.0	♥	
Japanese somen, cooked	½ cup	115	25	0.2	♥	
Japanese Udon, cooked	½ cup	115	12	0.3	♥	
plain, all types	½ cup	106	20	1.2	♥	
spinach, all types	½ cup	106	20	1.3	♥	T
Oats, cooked, see our Cereal section						

♥ = HEALTHY HEART FOOD   T = TRIGGER FOOD

Item	SERVING	CAL-ORIES	CARBS (g)	TOTAL FAT(g)	♥	T
Pasta						
protein-fortified	½ cup	115	22	0.2	♥	T
regular	½ cup	99	20	0.5	♥	T
spinach	½ cup	106	22	0.5	♥	T
whole wheat	½ cup	99	22	0.4	♥	T
Rice						
basmati	½ cup	115	22	0.5	♥	
brown						
long grain	½ cup	110	23	0.0	♥	
medium grain, precooked	½ cup	90	21	1.0	♥	
short grain	½ cup	115	25	0.5	♥	T
glutinous	½ cup	117	25	0.3	♥	
pilaf	½ cup	110	21	1.0	♥	
Spanish style, Birds Eye	½ cup	134	29	0.0	♥	
white	½ cup	113	25	0.0	♥	
white & wild, Green Giant frozen	½ cup	130	24	2.0	♥	
white, instant	½ cup	90	20	0.0	♥	
white, long grain	½ cup	100	22	0.0	♥	
white, medium grain	½ cup	133	29	0.2	♥	
wild rice	½ cup	83	18	0.0	♥	
Spaghetti						
cooked firm	½ cup	95	20	0.5	♥	T
cooked tender	½ cup	78	16	0.5	♥	T
Tabbouleh	½ cup	161	17	10.0		T

SALAD BAR AND DRESSINGS

Item	SERVING	CAL-ORIES	CARBS (g)	TOTAL FAT(g)	♥	T

Note: Portions in this section are for typical salad bar servings. For other vegetables and larger portions, see our Vegetable section.

Item	SERVING	CAL-ORIES	CARBS (g)	TOTAL FAT(g)	♥	T
Salad Bar Choices						
Alfalfa sprouts	¼ cup	2	0	0.0	♥	
Bacon bits	¼ cup	132	8	4.0		
Bean sprouts	¼ cup	8	2	0.2	♥	
Beets	¼ cup	18	4	0.1	♥	
Broccoli	¼ cup	6	1	0.1	♥	T
Cabbage	¼ cup	5	1	0.1	♥	
Cantaloupe	¼ cup	14	3	0.1	♥	

♥ = HEALTHY HEART FOOD   T = TRIGGER FOOD

Item	SERVING	CAL-ORIES	CARBS (g)	TOTAL FAT(g)	♥	T
Carrots	¼ cup	12	3	0.1	♥	T
Cauliflower	¼ cup	6	1	0.1	♥	
Cheddar cheese	¼ cup	100	0	8.0		
Chick-peas	¼ cup	55	9	1.0	♥	T
Chinese noodles	¼ cup	55	7	3.0		
Cottage cheese	¼ cup	58	2	2.0		T
Croutons	¼ cup	28	6	0.2	♥	
Cucumber	¼ cup	3	1	0.0	♥	
Dressings, see section that follows						
Egg, chopped	¼ cup	110	2	8.0		
Fruit cocktail	¼ cup	46	12	0.1	♥	
Garbanzo beans	¼ cup	55	9	1.0	♥	T
Gelatin parfait	¼ cup	50	10	2.0		
Granola	¼ cup	65	9	3.0		T
Greek pasta salad	¼ cup	159	19	9.0		
Green peas	¼ cup	28	5	0.1	♥	
Green pepper	¼ cup	6	2	0.2		
Honeydew	¼ cup	15	4	0.1	♥	
Lettuce						
iceberg	¼ cup	2	0	0.0	♥	
romaine	¼ cup	2	0	0.1	♥	
Macaroni salad	¼ cup	93	10	5.0		
Onions, chopped	¼ cup	14	4	0.2	♥	T
Peach	¼ cup	48	13	0.1	♥	T
Peas	¼ cup	28	5	0.1	♥	T
Pineapple chunks						
canned	¼ cup	48	12	0.1	♥	
fresh	¼ cup	19	5	0.1	♥	T
Potato salad	¼ cup	54	5	3.0		
Radish	¼ cup	4	2	0.2		
Strawberries, fresh	¼ cup	11	3	0.1	♥	T
Taco chips	1 oz.	186	29	7.1		
Taco shell	1	45	6	3.0		
Tomatoes	¼ cup	13	3	0.0	♥	T
Watermelon	¼ cup	13	3	0.1	♥	T
Salad Dressings						
Bacon & tomato, Kraft	1 Tbsp.	70	1	7.0		
Blue cheese						
low-calorie, Kraft chunky	1 Tbsp.	30	2	2.0		T
low-calorie, Roka	1 Tbsp.	16	1	1.0		T
regular, Kraft chunky	1 Tbsp.	60	2	6.0		
Caesar	1 Tbsp.	77	1	8.0		
Coleslaw dressing	1 Tbsp.	70	3	6.0		T

♥ = HEALTHY HEART FOOD   T = TRIGGER FOOD

Item	SERVING	CAL-ORIES	CARBS (g)	TOTAL FAT(g)	♥	T
Creamy cucumber, Kraft	1 Tbsp.	70	1	8.0		
Creamy Italian						
low-calorie	1 Tbsp.	26	2	2.0		T
regular	1 Tbsp.	56	2	5.5		
Dijon vinaigrette						
low-calorie	1 Tbsp.	30	1	2.8		T
regular	1 Tbsp.	60	1	6.1		
French						
low-calorie	1 Tbsp.	25	2	2.0		T
regular	1 Tbsp.	85	1	9.0		
garlic						
creamy	1 Tbsp.	74	1	8.0		
regular	1 Tbsp.	55	2	5.3		
Italian						
low-calorie	1 Tbsp.	5	2	0.0	♥	T
regular	1 Tbsp.	80	0	9.0		
Mayonnaise, Miracle Whip						
light	1 Tbsp.	45	2	4.0		T
regular	1 Tbsp.	70	2	7.0		
Onion & chives, Kraft creamy	1 Tbsp.	70	1	7.0		
Ranch	1 Tbsp.	78	1	8.3		
Russian						
low-calorie	1 Tbsp.	30	4	1.0		T
regular	1 Tbsp.	60	4	5.0		
Thousand Island						
low-calorie	1 Tbsp.	25	2	2.0		T
regular	1 Tbsp.	60	2	6.0		
Vinegar & oil	1 Tbsp.	75	0	8.0		
Vinegar & oil dressing, Kraft	1 Tbsp.	60	4	4.0		

SEAFOOD

Item	SERVING	CAL-ORIES	CARBS (g)	TOTAL FAT(g)	♥	T
Note: All values are for foods that are baked, broiled, or poached unless otherwise indicated.						
Albalone, canned	3 oz.	69	5	0.4	♥	
Anchovy, canned in oil, drained	3 oz.	180	0	8.4		
Bass, freshwater	3 oz.	90	0	3.0		

♥ = HEALTHY HEART FOOD   T = TRIGGER FOOD

Item	SERVING	CAL-ORIES	CARBS (g)	TOTAL FAT(g)	♥	T
Bluefish	3 oz.	105	0	3.6		
Butterfish	3 oz.	123	0	6.9		
Carp	3 oz.	138	0	6.0		
Catfish, breaded	3 oz.	195	6	12.0		
Caviar, jarred, black or red	3 oz.	213	3	15.0		
Clam						
boiled or steamed	3 oz.	126	3	1.8	♥	
breaded	3 oz.	171	9	9.6		
canned	3 oz.	126	3	1.8	♥	
Cod						
baked or broiled	3 oz.	90	0	0.9	♥	
canned w/liquid	3 oz.	90	0	0.9	♥	
Crab						
Alaska King						
boiled or steamed	3 oz.	84	0	1.2	♥	
canned	3 oz.	84	0	1.2	♥	
blue						
broiled	3 oz.	87	0	1.5	♥	
fried cake	3 oz.	132	0	6.3		
Crab, imitation	3 oz.	87	9	1.2	♥	T
Crayfish	3 oz.	75	0	0.9	♥	
Croaker, breaded or fried	3 oz.	189	9	10.8		
Dolphinfish	3 oz.	82	0	0.6	♥	
Eel, baked, broiled, or smoked	3 oz.	201	0	22.0		
Gefilte Fish						
in jellied broth	1 piece	210	15	3.0	♥	T
sweet w/broth	1 piece	72	6	1.5	♥	T
Grouper	3 oz.	102	0	1.2	♥	
Haddock						
baked or broiled	3 oz.	96	0	0.9	♥	
smoked	3 oz.	99	0	0.9	♥	
Halibut	3 oz.	119	0	1.8	♥	
Herring						
baked or broiled	3 oz.	174	0	9.9		
pickled	3 oz.	222	9	15.3		T
Lobster, boiled or steamed	3 oz.	84	0	0.6	♥	
Lox	3 oz.	99	0	3.6		
Lox, imitation (Mox Lox)	3 oz.	50	6	1.6		T
Mackerel						
baked or broiled	3 oz.	223	0	15.2		
canned	3 oz.	132	0	1.6	♥	
Mullet	3 oz.	99	0	3.3		
Mussel, boiled or steamed	3 oz.	146	6	3.8		
Ocean Perch	3 oz.	103	0	1.8	♥	

♥ = HEALTHY HEART FOOD   T = TRIGGER FOOD

Item	SERVING	CAL-ORIES	CARBS (g)	TOTAL FAT(g)	♥	T
Oyster						
boiled or steamed	3 oz.	117	6	4.2		
breaded & fried	3 oz.	168	9	10.8		
Perch	3 oz.	99	0	0.9	♥	
Pike	3 oz.	96	0	0.9	♥	
Pollack	3 oz.	78	0	0.8	♥	
Rockfish	3 oz.	102	0	1.8	♥	
Roe	3 oz.	120	0	5.4		
Sablefish, smoked	3 oz.	165	0	12.9		
Salmon						
baked, broiled or poached	3 oz.	184	0	9.3		
canned, in water	3 oz.	111	0	4.6		
kipper	3 oz.	165	0	12.9		
smoked (lox)	3 oz.	99	0	3.6		
Salmon, smoked, imitation	3 oz.	50	6	1.6		T
Sardines, canned						
in oil, drained	3 oz.	180	0	9.9		
in mustard sauce	3 oz.	176	2	12.8		
in tomato sauce, drained	3 oz.	176	2	12.8		
in water	3 oz.	139	1	10.2		
Sashimi	3 oz.	101	6	3.4		T
Scallops, breaded & fried	3 oz.	183	9	9.3		
Scallops, imitation	3 oz.	84	9	0.3	♥	T
Scrod	3 oz.	90	0	0.9	♥	
Sea bass	3 oz.	105	0	2.1	♥	
Shark, batter dipped	3 oz.	194	5	11.8		
Shrimp						
boiled, poached, or steamed	3 oz.	84	0	0.9	♥	
breaded and fried	3 oz.	207	9	10.5		
Shrimp, imitation	3 oz.	87	8	1.2	♥	T
Shrimp cocktail, Sau-Sea	4 oz.	113	19	1.0	♥	T
Shrimp salad (3 oz. scoop)						
commercial	3 oz.	126	6	9.0		T
homemade	3 oz.	128	1	9.0		
Sushi	3 oz.	101	6	3.4		T
Trout	3 oz.	129	0	0.9	♥	
Tuna						
baked or broiled	3 oz.	156	0	5.4		
canned in water, drained	3 oz.	111	0	0.3	♥	
canned in vegetable oil, drained	3 oz.	168	0	6.9		
Tuna, imitation	3 oz.	150	5	11.5		T
Tuna salad (3 oz. scoop)						

♥ = HEALTHY HEART FOOD   T = TRIGGER FOOD

Item	SERVING	CAL-ORIES	CARBS (g)	TOTAL FAT(g)	♥	T
commercial	3 oz.	174	9	12.0		T
homemade	3 oz.	170	1	11.0		
Turbot	3 oz.	81	0	2.4		
Whitefish, smoked	3 oz.	93	0	0.9	♥	
Whiting	3 oz.	99	0	1.5	♥	

SNACK FOODS, CHIPS, AND DIPS

Item	SERVING	CAL-ORIES	CARBS (g)	TOTAL FAT(g)	♥	T
Note: For sweet snacks such as candy, cake, donuts, and cookies, see our Sweets, Desserts, and Toppings section.						
Bagel chips						
cinnamon raisin	1 oz.	130	18	5.0		T
garlic	1 oz.	150	15	9.0		
hot & spicy	1 oz.	135	17	5.0		T
onion	1 oz.	150	15	9.0		
Bugles						
nacho	1 oz.	160	19	9.0		
regular	1 oz.	160	18	8.0		
Cheese puffs						
Cheetos	1 oz.	160	15	10.0		
Cheez Balls, Planters	1 oz.	160	14	11.0		
Chips						
baked chips						
multigrain, Sun Chips	1 oz.	140	18	7.0		T
regular, Zings	1 oz.	140	18	6.0		
Corn chips						
nacho, Doritos	1 oz.	140	18	7.0		
plain						
Fritos	1 oz.	150	16	9.0		
most brands	1 oz.	155	16	9.0		
Pringle's	1 oz.	140	17	7.0		
Wise	1 oz.	160	15	10.0		
tortilla, Dorito's	1 oz.	140	19	6.0		
Potato chips						
barbecue flavor						
Bachman	1 oz.	150	14	9.0		
Wise	1 oz.	150	14	10.0		
cheese, Pringle's	1 oz.	170	12	13.0		

♥ = HEALTHY HEART FOOD   T = TRIGGER FOOD

Item	SERVING	CAL-ORIES	CARBS (g)	TOTAL FAT(g)	♥	T
onion-garlic, Wise	1 oz.	150	14	10.0		
plain						
Bachman Kettle Cooked	1 oz.	140	16	8.0		
Pringle's original	1 oz.	170	12	13.0		
sour cream & onion						
Pringle's	1 oz.	150	14	11.0		
Ruffles	1 oz.	150	15	9.0		
Potato skins, Tato skins	1 oz.	150	17	8.0		
Combos						
cheese	1 oz.	147	16	8.2		
peanut butter	1 oz.	133	17	5.6		
pizza	1 oz.	141	18	6.5		
Corn dog	1	330	27	20.0		
Crackers, see our Breads, Crackers, and Flour section						
Cracker Jack	1 oz.	120	22	3.0		
Dips						
avocado	1 Tbsp.	25	2	2.0		
bacon & horseradish	1 Tbsp.	30	2	2.5		T
bacon & onion	1 Tbsp.	35	1	3.0		
blue cheese	1 Tbsp.	25	1	2.0		
chili	1 Tbsp.	6	1	0.6		
clam	1 Tbsp.	30	2	2.0		T
nacho	1 Tbsp.	28	1	2.0		
onion	1 Tbsp.	30	2	2.0		T
French fried onions, canned Durkee	1 oz.	160	10	12.0		
Fruit snacks						
Delmonte yogurt raisins	1 pouch	120	18	5.0		T
Dinosaurs	1 pouch	90	21	1.0	♥	T
Fruit rocks	1 pouch	100	22	1.0	♥	T
Fruit rolls, all flavors	1	50	12	1.0	♥	T
Garfield	1 pouch	100	22	1.0	♥	
Shark bits	1 pouch	100	22	1.0	♥	
Sharks	1 pouch	90	21	1.0	♥	
Sunkist Fun Fruits	1 pouch	100	22	1.4	♥	T
Tail spin	1 pouch	100	22	1.0	♥	T
Goldfish, all varieties	1 oz.	120	9	3.0		
Party mix, see snack mix in this section						
Pita chips, all flavors	1 oz.	133	19	4.0		T
Popcorn						
air popped	3 cups	90	18	0.0	♥	T
microwaved, butter flavor						
Joly Time	3 cups	150	18	7.0		

♥ = HEALTHY HEART FOOD   T = TRIGGER FOOD

Item	SERVING	CAL-ORIES	CARBS (g)	TOTAL FAT(g)	♥	T
Planters	3 cups	140	13	10.0		
microwaved, cheese, Jolly Time	3 cups	180	17	11.0		
microwaved, plain						
Jolly Time	3 cups	150	15	10.0		T
Pillsbury Original	3 cups	210	20	13.0		
packaged, pre-popped						
cheese, Smartfood	1 oz.	160	14	10.0		
plain, Frito-Lay	1 oz.	140	18	6.0		T
sugar coated, Cracker Jacks	1 oz.	120	22	3.0		
Pork rind snack	1 oz.	160	2	10.0		
Potato sticks	1 oz.	140	16	8.0		
Pretzels						
beer	1 oz.	110	24	1.0	♥	
logs	1 oz.	103	22	0.8	♥	
thin rings, twists, sticks	1 oz.	110	21	2.0	♥	
Pringle's, see Chips, Potato chips						
Rice cakes						
Chico San						
cinnamon crunch	1	60	9	2.0		T
popcorn	1	50	10	2.0		T
ranch style	1	50	8	2.0		
Quaker, all varieties	1	35	7	0.3	♥	T
Pacific Grain, apple cinnamon	1	35	7	1.0	♥	T
Sesame buds	1 oz.	165	11	12.0		T
Snack Bars						
Kudos, nutty fudge/peanut butter	1	200	20	12.0		
Nature Valley, oat bran granola	1	110	16	4.0		T
Nutri-Grain, cereal bars	1	150	25	5.0		T
Oat bran, date-almond bar	1	140	27	2.0	♥	T
Quaker granola, all flavors	1	125	19	5.0		T
Rice Crispy	1	120	21	4.0		
Snack Mixes						
Chex Mix, Ralston original	1 oz.	110	16	4.0		
Eagle Snack Mix	1 oz.	140	18	6.0		
Love Snacks						
Ambrosia	1 oz.	110	22	2.0	♥	T
Athletes' Mix	1 oz.	140	14	8.0		T
Fruit & Nut	1 oz.	150	11	10.0		T
Nutty Mix	1 oz.	150	11	10.0		T

♥ = HEALTHY HEART FOOD   T = TRIGGER FOOD

Item	SERVING	CAL-ORIES	CARBS (g)	TOTAL FAT(g)	♥	T
Raisin & Cashew	1 oz.	110	18	14.0	♥	T
Tropical Mix	1 oz.	120	16	5.0		T
Yogurt Trail Mix	1 oz.	120	17	0.5	♥	T
Party mix, Flavor Tree	1 oz.	160	10	11.0		
Pepperidge Farm mix, smoked	1 oz.	150	13	9.0		

SOUPS

Item	SERVING	CAL-ORIES	CARBS (g)	TOTAL FAT(g)	♥	T
Bean						
bean only	1 cup	192	32	3.2	♥	T
w/bacon	1 cup	144	24	4.0		
w/ham	1 cup	160	24	3.2	♥	
Beef	1 cup	136	16	4.8		T
Beef bouillon	1 cup	15	0	1.0		T
Beef broth	1 cup	15	0	1.0		T
Beef consommé	1 cup	15	0	1.0		T
Beef minestrone	1 cup	144	16	4.0		
Beef noodle	1 cup	85	9	3.0		
Beef noodle, Progresso	1 cup	144	16	3.2		
Beef w/bacon	1 cup	170	23	6.0		
Beef w/vegetables & pasta	1 cup	104	16	1.6	♥	
Beef Stroganoff	1 cup	240	24	12.0		
Borscht	1 cup	104	24	0.0	♥	T
Chicken	1 cup	96	8	2.4		T
Chicken broth	1 cup	32	0	3.2		T
Chicken corn chowder	1 cup	256	16	16.0		
Chicken gumbo w/sausage	1 cup	104	8	2.4		
Chicken creamy mushroom	1 cup	200	8	14.4		
Chicken noodle						
Campbell's Chunky	1 cup	152	16	5.6		
canned	1 cup	75	9	2.0		
from mix	1 pkt.	40	6	1.0		
Chicken rice	1 cup	60	7	2.0		
Chicken rice, Campbell's Home Cookin'	1 cup	112	8	4.0		
Clam chowder						
Manhattan style	1 cup	80	12	2.0		
Manhattan style, Progresso	1 cup	104	8	1.6	♥	
New England style	1 cup	165	17	7.0		

♥ = HEALTHY HEART FOOD   T = TRIGGER FOOD

Item	SERVING	CAL-ORIES	CARBS (g)	TOTAL FAT(g)	♥	T
New England style, Progresso	1 cup	192	16	10.4		
Cream of celery	1 cup	104	8	7.2		
Cream of chicken						
made w/milk	1 cup	190	15	11.0		
made w/water	1 cup	115	9	7.0		
Cream of mushroom						
made w/milk	1 cup	205	15	14.0		
made w/water	1 cup	130	9	9.0		
Cream of tomato	1 cup	112	24	3.2		
French onion						
canned, w/o cheese	1 cup	64	8	2.4		T
from mix	1 pkt.	20	4	0.0	♥	T
Ham and bean	1 cup	120	24	1.6	♥	
Lentil	1 cup	120	24	3.2		
Minestrone	1 cup	80	11	3.0		
Minestrone, Progresso	1 cup	112	16	3.2		
Split pea w/ham	1 cup	176	24	4.0		
Tomato						
made w/milk	1 cup	160	22	6.0		
made w/water	1 cup	85	17	2.0		
Tomato vegetable, from mix	1 pkt.	40	8	1.0		
Turkey vegetable	1 cup	128	16	4.8		
Vegetable	1 cup	88	16	2.4		
Vegetable beef	1 cup	80	10	2.0		
Vegetarian beef	1 cup	70	12	2.0		T
Won Ton	1 cup	40	8	0.8	♥	T

SWEETS, DESSERTS, AND TOPPINGS

Item	SERVING	CAL-ORIES	CARBS (g)	TOTAL FAT(g)	♥	T

Note: Average servings noted below are usually equal to about 1/12 of a larger cake or 1/8 of a good-sized pie. They are equal to a typical restaurant portion or, if the food is packaged, as indicated on the package.

Item	SERVING	CAL-ORIES	CARBS (g)	TOTAL FAT(g)	♥	T
Apple butter	1 tsp.	12	3	0.0	♥	T
Breath mints						
Breath Savers, spearmint	1	8	2	0.0	♥	T
Clorets	1	6	2	0.0	♥	T
Tic Tac	1	2	0	0.0	♥	T

♥ = HEALTHY HEART FOOD   T = TRIGGER FOOD

Item	SERVING	CAL-ORIES	CARBS (g)	TOTAL FAT(g)	♥	T
Brownie w/nuts & frosting	1 serv.	100	14	5.0		
Cake						
angel food						
from mix	1 serv.	130	30	0.0	♥	
homemade	1 serv.	125	29	0.0	♥	
apple streusel	1 serv.	160	18	9.0		
banana, iced	1 serv.	140	17	8.0		
black forest						
frozen, Sara Lee	1 serv.	190	28	8.0		
blueberry crunch, Entenmann's	1 serv.	70	16	0.0	♥	
Boston cream						
frozen	1 serv.	290	39	14.0		
homemade	1 serv.	270	50	6.0		
butter pecan	1 serv.	250	35	11.0		
carrot						
from mix	1 serv.	250	35	11.0		
frozen w/icing, Pepperidge Farm	1 serv.	150	19	9.0		
homemade w/icing	1 serv.	385	48	21.0		
cheese						
cherry, frozen	1 serv.	243	35	8.0		
French, frozen	1 serv.	250	23	16.0		
plain						
from mix	1 serv.	280	36	13.0		
frozen	1 serv.	230	27	11.0		
strawberry, frozen	1 serv.	222	34	8.0		
cheese substitute, nondairy	1 serv.	280	26	18.0		
chocolate						
frozen, Sara Lee Free & Lite	1 serv.	110	26	0.0	♥	
homemade	1 serv.	250	38	11.0		
chocolate fudge, from mix	1 serv.	260	34	12.0		
chocolate mousse, frozen	1 serv.	260	23	17.0		
coconut	1 serv.	160	19	9.0		
coffee cake						
caramel nut	1 serv.	140	15	8.0		
cheese	1 serv.	210	25	11.0		
pecan, Sara Lee	1 serv.	160	19	8.0		
streusel, Sara Lee	1 serv.	160	20	7.0		
cream cheese, see Cake, cheese						
devil's food						
from mix	1 serv.	260	35	12.0		
homemade	1 serv.	235	40	8.0		

♥ = HEALTHY HEART FOOD   T = TRIGGER FOOD

Item	SERVING	CAL-ORIES	CARBS (g)	TOTAL FAT(g)	♥	T
w/cream filling	1 serv.	105	17	4.0		
fruitcake, dark	1 serv.	165	25	7.0		
gingerbread	1 serv.	175	32	4.0		
lemon, three layer	1 serv.	320	38	5.0	♥	
Neopolitan torte	1 serv.	380	43	22.0		
orange w/icing	1 serv.	150	19	8.0		
peanut butter torte	1 serv.	380	44	22.0		
pineapple crunch, Entenmann's	1 serv.	70	16	0.0	♥	
pound						
frozen	1 serv.	110	13	6.0		T
homemade	1 serv.	130	19	5.0		T
sheet cake						
w/frosting	1 serv.	445	77	14.0		
w/o frosting	1 serv	315	48	12.0		T
sponge						
creme filled	1 serv.	155	27	5.0		
w/o filling	1 serv.	80	11	3.0		T
streusel, apple	1 serv.	160	18	9.0		
walnut torte	1 serv.	320	28	19.0		
white						
from mix	1 serv.	240	37	9.0		
homemade	1 serv.	270	34	15.0		
yellow						
from mix	1 serv.	260	36	11.0		
homemade	1 serv.	290	33	17.0		
Cake, snack						
apple, Hostess Light	1 piece	130	29	1.0	♥	
banana, Hostess Twinkies	1 piece	150	26	5.0		
Boston cream pie, frozen	1 serv.	230	34	10.0		
carrot, frozen	1 serv.	260	32	16.0		
cheesecake, strawberry, frozen	1 serv.	300	49	9.0		
Choco Bliss	1 piece	200	29	9.0		
Choco-Diles	1 piece	240	32	11.0		
Creamie	1 piece	184	25	9.0		
Ding Dongs	1 piece	170	21	9.0		
Drake's Jr. coffee cake	1 piece	140	18	6.0		
Hi-Ho's	1 piece	120	16	6.0		
Hostess, chocolate	1 piece	180	30	6.0		
Hostess Light, cream-filled chocolate	1 piece	130	26	2.0	♥	
Kandy Kakes, peanut butter	1 piece	87	11	4.2		
Koffee Kake, cream filled	1 piece	110	18	4.0		

♥ = HEALTHY HEART FOOD   T = TRIGGER FOOD

Item	SERVING	CAL-ORIES	CARBS (g)	TOTAL FAT(g)	♥	T
Koffee Kake Jrs.	1 piece	261	44	8.5		
Krimpets, cream-filled	1 piece	124	20	4.3		
Krimpets, jelly-filled	1 piece	85	19	1.0	♥	
Pecan twirls	1 piece	109	17	4.9		
Pepperidge Farm, double chocolate, frozen	1 serv.	250	31	13.0		
Ring-Dings, Drakes, cream-filled	1 piece	100	16	4.0		
Sara Lee, fudge, frozen	1 serv.	190	24	10.0		
Suzy Q's	1 piece	250	37	10.0		
Tandy Takes, Tastykake	1 piece	78	12	3.1		
Tastykake chocolate snack cake	1 piece	100	19	2.6		
Tastylite, cream-filled chocolate	1 piece	100	22	1.3	♥	
Twinkies, creme-filled	1 piece	150	27	5.0		
Twinkies Fruit N Creme	1 piece	140	27	3.0	♥	
Twinkies Light, creme-filled	1 piece	110	21	2.0	♥	
Candy						
Almond Joy	1 oz.	142	16	8.0		
Baby Ruth	1 oz.	130	18	6.0		
Bit-O-Honey	1 oz.	118	23	2.4	♥	
Butterfinger	1 oz.	130	19	6.0		
candy canes	1 oz.	110	27	0.0	♥	
caramels, plain/chocolate	1 oz.	115	22	3.0		
Charleston Chew!	1 oz.	120	22	3.0		
chocolate bars						
dark chocolate	1 oz.	150	16	10.0		
Kit Kat	1 oz.	153	18.0	8.0		
Mars bar	1 oz.	136	17	6.3		
milk chocolate, plain, Hershey's	1 oz.	155	16	9.0		
milk chocolate w/almonds, Hershey's	1 oz.	159	14	9.7		
milk chocolate w/peanuts	1 oz.	155	13	11.0		
milk chocolate w/rice cereal	1 oz.	10	18	7.0		
Milky Way	1 oz.	130	20	5.1		
Milky Way, dark	1 oz.	125	20	4.5		
Mounds	1 oz.	137	16	7.4		
Mr. Goodbar	1 oz.	166	13	10.9		
Nestlé Crunch	1 oz.	150	19	7.1		
Snickers	1 oz.	135	17	6.8		
3 Musketeers	1 oz.	122	22	3.8		

♥ = HEALTHY HEART FOOD   T = TRIGGER FOOD

Item	SERVING	CAL-ORIES	CARBS (g)	TOTAL FAT(g)	♥	T
chocolate-covered pea-nuts	1 oz.	150	15	9.0		
chocolate-covered raisins	1 oz.	130	20	5.0		
chocolate Santa	1 oz.	140	18	7.0		
cough drops, see our Medications section						
Creme de Menthe, Brach's	1 oz.	150	16	9.0		
creme egg, Brach's	1 oz.	110	23	2.0	♥	
creme egg, Cadbury	1 oz.	139	19	5.8	♥	
fondant	1 oz.	105	27	0.0	♥	
fudge	1 oz.	115	21	3.0		
Good & Fruity	1 oz.	106	26	0.1	♥	
Good & Plenty	1 oz.	106	26	0.0	♥	
gum, see Gum (below) in this section						
gumdrops	1 oz.	100	25	0.0	♥	
Gummy Bears	1 oz.	100	22	0.0	♥	
hard candy						
regular	1 oz.	110	28	0.0	♥	T
Hide'n Seek eggs, Brach's	1 oz.	110	27	0.0	♥	
Indian corn, Brach's	1 oz.	100	26	0.0	♥	
Jellies, Brach's	1 oz.	100	24	0.0	♥	
jelly beans	1 oz.	100	26	0.0		
Jujyfruits	1 oz.	100	25	0.7	♥	
Junior Mints	1 oz.	120	24	3.0		
Kit Kat	1 oz.	153	18	8.0		
Life Savers, all flavors	1 oz.	110	28	0.0	♥	T
M&M's	1 oz.	148	20	7.1		
malted milk balls	1 oz.	130	21	5.0		
marshmallows	1 oz.	25	6	0.0		
marshmallow Santa	1 oz.	120	23	3.0		
Milk Maid, Brach's	1 oz.	110	20	3.0		
Nut Goodies, Brach's	1 oz.	130	21	4.0		
Ornaments, Brach's	1 oz.	150	17	8.0		
Parfait, Brach's	1 oz.	150	16	9.0		
peanut brittle	1 oz.	130	20	5.0		
Pom Poms	1 oz.	100	15	3.0		
Pumpkins, Brach's	1 oz.	100	26	0.0	♥	
Raisinets	1 oz.	131	20	4.4		
Reese's Pieces	1 oz.	141	17	5.9		
saltwater taffy	1 oz.	100	24	1.0	♥	
Scary Cats, Brach's	1 oz.	100	26	0.0	♥	
Sno-Caps	1 oz.	140	21	6.0		
sour balls	1 oz.	110	27	0.0	♥	T
spearmint leaves	1 oz.	100	24	0.0	♥	
Speckled jelly, Brach's	1 oz.	110	27	0.0	♥	

♥ = HEALTHY HEART FOOD   T = TRIGGER FOOD

Item	SERVING	CAL-ORIES	CARBS (g)	TOTAL FAT(g)	♥	T
Starburst	1 oz.	116	23	2.4	♥	
Sugarless candies*						
Toffy, Brach's	1 oz.	110	23	2.0	♥	
Trick or Treat pack, Brach's	1 oz.	110	26	0.0	♥	
Tootsie Roll	1 oz.	112	23	2.5		
Valentine's Day heart, Brach's	1 oz.	110	23	0.0	♥	
Valentine's Day, I Luv U, Brach's	1 oz.	150	17	8.0		
Valentine's Day, Mellowcremes	1 oz.	100	26	0.0	♥	
Y&S Twizzlers, strawberry	1 oz.	100	23	1.0	♥	
York Peppermint Patties	1 oz.	120	23	2.7		
Cookies						
animal crackers	1	20	2	0.4	♥	
Anisette Sponge	1	51	10	0.8	♥	
Anisette Toast	1	46	9	0.6	♥	
Anisette Toast, Jumbo	1	109	23	1.0	♥	
Apple Newtons	1	80	15	2.0		
Apple n'raisin	1	120	20	3.0		
Arrowroot biscuit	1	20	3	1.0		
Baby Bear, Keebler	1	23	3	1.0		
Beacon Hill, Pepperidge Farm	1	120	14	7.0		
Bordeaux Pepperidge Farm	1	35	6	1.5		
Breakfast Treats, Stella D'oro	1	101	15	3.6		
Brownie, Pepperidge Farm	1	55	6	3.5		
Brussels, Pepperidge Farm	1	55	7	2.5		
Brussels Mint, Pepperidge Farm	1	65	8	3.5		
Cappuccino, Pepperidge Farm	1	50	6	3.0		
Capri, Pepperidge Farm	1	80	10	5.0		
Carrot walnut	1	60	11	1.0	♥	
Castelets, Stella D'oro	1	64	9	2.8		
Chantilly, Pepperidge Farm	1	80	14	2.0		
Chesapeake, chocolate chip/chunk	1	120	14	7.0		

♥ = HEALTHY HEART FOOD   T = TRIGGER FOOD
*Sugarless candies vary in caloric and fat contents, and their labeling makes comparisons difficult. "Sugarless" candies contain no sucrose, but they are usually high in other sugars and carbohydrates. They will often trigger cravings for additional sweets and other carbohydrates.

Item	SERVING	CAL-ORIES	CARBS (g)	TOTAL FAT(g)	♥	T
Chessman, Pepperidge Farm	1	45	6	2.0		
Cheyenne, Pepperidge Farm	1	110	13	6.0		
Chinese almond cookies	1	169	20	8.9		
chocolate cookies						
Snaps, chocolate fudge	1	18	3	0.5		
Swiss, Stella D'oro	1	68	9	3.4		
chocolate chip/chunk						
homemade	1	50	7	3.0		
Almost Home Real	1	60	7	3.0		
chewy Chips Ahoy!	1	60	7	3.0		
Grandma's Big Cookies	1	185	25	8.5		
Keebler Deluxe	1	80	10	4.0		
Stella D'oro Swiss	1	68	9	3.4		
Tastykake Bar	1	211	35	7.7		
chocolate sandwich	1	49	7	2.0		
Dutch Bar, apple	1	112	19	3.3		
egg biscuit	1	43	7	1.1		
E. L. Fudge, Keebler	1	40	5	2.0		
Fig Newton	1	60	11	1.0	♥	
French Vanilla Creme, Keebler	1	80	12	4.0		
Fruit cookies, Pepperidge Farm	1	50	8	2.0		
Fudge Sticks, Keebler	1	50	7	2.5		
Fudge Stripes, Keebler	1	50	7	3.0		
Geneva, Pepperidge Farm	1	65	7	3.0		
gingersnaps						
Archway	1	35	6	1.0		
Nabisco Old Fashioned	1	30	6	1.0		
Golden bars, Stella D'oro	1	109	16	4.3		
Graham cracker						
cinnamon, Keebler Crisp	1	18	3	0.5		
honey	1	30	6	0.5	♥	
plain, Keebler	1	18	3	0.5		T
Granola sandwich, Incredibites	1 pouch	170	24	7.0		
Granola bars, see our Snacks section						
Grasshopper, Keebler	1	35	5	1.5		
Lido, Pepperidge Farm	1	90	10	5.0		
Lorna Doone	1	23	3	1.0		
macaroon	1	60	7	3.4		

Item	SERVING	CAL-ORIES	CARBS (g)	TOTAL FAT(g)	♥	T
Magic Middles, chocolate w/chocolate chip	1	80	9	5.0		
Mallowmars	1	60	9	3.0		
Mandel Toasts, Stella D'oro	1	58	10	1.4		T
Margherite, Stella D'oro	1	72	10	3.1		
Milano Mint, Pepperidge Farm	1	75	8	3.5		
Milano Orange, Pepperidge Farm	1	75	8	3.5		
Milano, Pepperidge Farm	1	60	8	3.0		
Mystic Mint	1	90	11	5.0		
Nantucket, Pepperidge Farm	1	120	15	6.0		
Nassau, Pepperidge Farm	1	80	9	5.0		
Nutter Butter sandwich	1	70	9	3.0		
Oat Bran Fruity Jumbo Health Valley	1	70	10	2.0		
oatmeal						
Archway	1	110	19	3.0		
Keebler Old Fashioned	1	80	12	3.0		
w/chocolate chunks, Chips Ahoy!	1	95	10	5.0		
Oreo	1	50	8	2.0		
Oreo Big Stuf	1	250	33	12.0		
Oreo Double Stuf	1	70	9	4.0		
Oreo, fudge covered	1	110	13	6.0		
peanut butter, Grandma's Big Cookies	1	205	22	15.0		
peanut butter	1	61	7	4.0		
pecan crunch, Archway	1	60	8	3.0		
Pecan Sandies, Keebler	1	80	9	5.0		
Pinwheels	1	103	20	5.0		
Pirouettes, Pepperidge Farm						
chocolate lace	1	35	4	2.0		
plain	1	35	4	2.0		
Raisin Bran, Pepperidge Farm	1	55	7	2.5		
Santa Fe, Pepperidge Farm	1	100	16	4.0		
Sausalito, Pepperidge Farm	1	120	14	7.0		
sesame	1	45	6	2.0		
shortbread						
homemade	1	50	6	4.0		
Pepperidge Farm, Old Fashioned	1	70	7	5.0		

♥ = HEALTHY HEART FOOD   T = TRIGGER FOOD

Item	SERVING	CAL-ORIES	CARBS (g)	TOTAL FAT(g)	♥	T
Strawberry Newton	1	120	23	3.0		
Suddenly S'Mores	1	100	15	4.0		
Sugar cookies						
homemade	1	25	4	1.0		
Pepperidge Farm	1	50	7	2.5		
Sugarless cookies*						T
Tahiti, Pepperidge Farm	1	90	9	6.0		
Teddy Grahams, chocolate covered	1	5	1	0.2		
Trolley Cakes	1	60	13	1.0	♥	
Twirls	1	140	20	6.0		
Vanilla wafers	1	19	3	0.7		
Venice, Pepperidge Farm	1	60	7	3.0		
Zurich, Pepperidge Farm	1	60	10	2.0		
Cupcakes						
Devil's food	1	120	20	4.0		
Devil's food w/icing	1	159	23	5.0		
Yellow w/icing	1	130	21	5.0		
Yellow w/o icing	1	90	14	3.0		
Custard, baked	1 serv.	305	29	15.0		
Danish pastry						
cheese	1	280	34	15.0		
fruit or nuts	1	235	28	13.0		
plain	1	220	26	12.0		
Donuts						
Bavarian filled, Dunkin' Donuts	1	240	32	11.0		
Blueberry filled, Dunkin' Donuts	1	210	29	8.0		
cake type	1	210	24	12.0		
cinnamon	1	140	14	8.0		
Coffee roll, glazed, Dunkin' donuts	1	280	37	12.0		
crumb	1	160	16	10.0		
French cruller, Dunkin' Donut	1	140	16	8.0		
frosted, vanilla	1	190	20	12.0		
glazed	1	250	33	12.0		
honey wheat	1	250	32	12.0		

♥ = HEALTHY HEART FOOD   T = TRIGGER FOOD
*Sugarless cookies vary in caloric and fat contents, and their labeling makes comparisons difficult. "Sugarless" cookies contain no sucrose, but they are usually high in other sugars and carbohydrates. They will often trigger cravings for additional sweets and other carbohydrates.

Item	SERVING	CAL-ORIES	CARBS (g)	TOTAL FAT(g)	♥	T
jelly filled, Dunkin' Donuts	1	220	31	9.0		
plain	1	145	13	6.0		
powdered sugar	1	150	16	8.0		
Food replacement bar						
Ultra Slim Fast, vanilla almond crunch	1 oz.	120	19	4.0		T
Gelatin						
D-Zerta, low-cal, all flavors	½ cup	8	0	0.0	♥	T
Jell-O, all flavors	½ cup	80	19	0.0	♥	T
Royal, all flavors	½ cup	80	19	0.0	♥	T
Gum						
Beechies	1 piece	6	2	0.0	♥	
Beech-Nut	1 piece	10	2	0.0	♥	
Big Red	1 piece	10	2	0.0	♥	
Bubble Yum	1 piece	25	7	0.0	♥	
Bubble Care Free	1 piece	10	2	0.0	♥	T
Bubblicious	1 piece	25	6	0.0	♥	
Care Free	1 piece	8	2	0.0	♥	T
Chewels	1 piece	8	2	0.0	♥	
Chiclets	1 piece	6	2	0.0	♥	T
Dentyne	1 piece	6	2	0.0	♥	
Dentyne, sugarless	1 piece	5	1	0.0	♥	T
Doublemint	1 piece	10	2	0.0	♥	
Freedent	1 piece	10	2	0.0	♥	T
Freshen-Up	1 piece	13	3	0.0	♥	
Hubba Bubba	1 piece	23	6	0.0	♥	
Juicy Fruit	1 piece	10	2	0.0	♥	T
Wrigley's Spearmint	1 piece	10	2	0.0	♥	T
Honey	1 tsp.	22	6	0.0	♥	T
Ice cream						
butter pecan						
hard						
Breyers	½ cup	180	15	12.0		
Häagen-Dazs	½ cup	390	29	24.0		
chocolate						
hard						
Breyers	½ cup	160	20	8.0		
Häagen-Dazs	½ cup	270	24	17.0		
soft	½ cup	194	7	12.0		
vanilla						
hard						
Breyers	½ cup	150	15	8.0		
Häagen Dazs	½ cup	260	23	17.0		
soft	½ cup	188	6	11.5		

♥ = HEALTHY HEART FOOD   T = TRIGGER FOOD

Item	SERVING	CAL-ORIES	CARBS (g)	TOTAL FAT(g)	♥	T
Ice cream substitute						
all flavors, Lite Lite Tofutti	½ cup	90	20	0.4	♥	T
chocolate, Sealtest Free	½ cup	100	23	0.0	♥	T
vanilla, Sealtest Free	½ cup	100	24	0.0	♥	T
vanilla, Tofutti	½ cup	200	21	11.0		T
Ice cream bars						
Good Humor						
chocolate fudge cake	1	214	18	15.0		
Halo Bar	1	230	23	13.7		
vanilla, chocolate-covered	1	198	17	13.7		
Klondike	1	280	23	19.0		
Ice cream bars, substitute						
chocolate fudge, Good Humor	1	127	27	0.6	♥	
Cool Shark, Good Humor	1	68	17	0.1	♥	
Ice cream cone, King Cone, Good Humor	1	290	41	12.0		
Ice cream sandwich	1	191	31	5.7		
Ice cream sandwich, substitute						
vanilla sandwich, Good Humor	1	150	28	3.0	♥	
Ice milk						
chocolate, hard, Borden	½ cup	100	18	2.0	♥	T
heavenly hash, Sealtest	½ cup	150	19	7.0		
vanilla, hard, Borden	½ cup	90	17	2.0		T
vanilla, soft	½ cup	113	19	2.5		T
Jams & preserves						
all flavors, Polaner	1 tsp.	18	5	0.0	♥	T
all flavors, Smucker's	1 tsp.	18	4	0.0	♥	
orange marmalade, Smucker's	1 tsp.	18	4	0.0	♥	
strawberry, Finast	1 tsp.	18	5	0.0	♥	
strawberry, imitation, Smucker's	1 tsp.	2	1	0.0	♥	
strawberry, low-calorie, Kraft	1 tsp.	6	2	0.0	♥	T
Jelly						
all flavors, Kraft	1 tsp.	17	4	0.0	♥	
all flavors, Smucker's	1 tsp.	18	4	0.0	♥	
grape, imitation, Smucker's	1 tsp.	2	1	0.0	♥	T
grape, low-calorie, Kraft	1 tsp.	6	2	0.0	♥	T
grape, Welch's	1 tsp.	18	5	0.0	♥	

♥ = HEALTHY HEART FOOD   T = TRIGGER FOOD

Item	SERVING	CAL-ORIES	CARBS (g)	TOTAL FAT(g)	♥	T
Muffin						
banana nut, Dunkin' Donuts	1	310	49	10.0		
blueberry						
Dunkin' Donuts*	1	280	46	8.0		
most commercial brands	1	140	21	5.0		
bran						
most commercial brands	1	135	21	6.0		
w/raisins, Dunkin' Do-nuts*	1	310	51	9.0		
corn						
Dunkin' Donuts*	1	340	51	12.0		
most commercial brands	1	145	22	6.0		
oat bran, Dunkin' Donuts*	1	330	50	11.0		
Pie						
apple						
fresh*	1 serv.	405	60	18.0		
frozen, Mrs. Smith's	1 serv.	210	29	9.0		
banana cream, frozen	1 serv.	180	21	10.0		
blueberry						
fresh*	1 serv.	380	55	17.0		
frozen Mrs. Smith's	1 serv.	220	32	9.0		
cherry						
fresh*	1 serv.	410	61	18.0		
frozen, Mrs. Smith's	1 serv.	220	32	9.0		
chocolate cream, frozen	1 serv.	190	24	10.0		
coconut cream, frozen	1 serv.	190	22	11.0		
cream	1 serv.	455	59	23.0		
cream cheese, see Cake, cheese						
custard	1 serv.	330	36	17.0		
lemon cream, frozen	1 serv.	170	23	9.0		
lemon meringue						
fresh*	1 serv.	335	53	14.0		
frozen, Mrs. Smith's	1 serv.	210	38	5.0		
peach						
fresh*	1 serv.	405	60	17.0		
frozen, Mrs. Smith's	1 serv.	210	29	9.0		
pecan						
fresh*	1 serv.	575	71	32.0		
frozen, Mrs. Smith's	1 serv.	330	51	13.0		
pumpkin						
fresh*	1 serv.	320	37	17.0		
frozen, Mrs. Smith's	1 serv.	190	30	6.0		

♥ = HEALTHY HEART FOOD   T = TRIGGER FOOD
*Higher caloric, carbohydrate, and fat contents may be due in whole or in part to larger portions per muffin or average serving.

Item	SERVING	CAL-ORIES	CARBS (g)	TOTAL FAT(g)	♥	T
strawberry, cream, frozen	I serv.	170	22	9.0		
Pies, snack						
apple, Hostess	I serv.	430	60	20.0		
apple, Tastykake	I serv.	296	46	12.3		
blackberry, Hostess	I serv.	420	59	18.0		
cherry, Hostess	I serv.	460	65	20.0		
lemon, Hostess	I serv.	440	60	20.0		
Popsicles						
most flavors	3 oz. pop.	70	18	0.0	♥	
Ice Stripes, all flavors	I bar	35	9	0.0	♥	
Pudding						
butterscotch	½ cup	120	25	4.0	♥	
chocolate	½ cup	155	26	4.0		
rice	½ cup	155	27	4.0		
tapioca	½ cup	145	25	4.0		
vanilla	½ cup	150	26	4.0		
Pudding pops, chocolate/ vanilla	I	80	13	2.0		
Snack cakes, see Cakes, snack, in this secion						
Sugar						
brown, light	I tsp.	12	3	0.0	♥	
white, granulated	I tsp.	14	4	0.0	♥	
white, granulated	I packet	25	6	0.0	♥	
Sherbet						
all flavors, Sealtest	½ cup	130	28	1.0	♥	T
most brands & flavors	½ cup	135	30	2.0	♥	T
Sorbet						
mandarin orange, Dole	½ cup	110	28	0.1	♥	T
raspberry, Dole	½ cup	110	28	0.1	♥	T
Syrup						
chocolate-flavored	I Tbsp.	43	11	0.0	♥	
corn	I Tbsp.	61	16	0.0	♥	
fudge	I Tbsp.	63	11	2.5		
maple	I Tbsp.	61	16	0.0	♥	
molasses	I Tbsp.	43	11	0.0	♥	
Toaster pastries	I	210	38	6.0		
Topping						
butterscotch	I Tbsp.	60	14	1.0	♥	
chocolate	I Tbsp.	50	11	0.0	♥	
chocolate fudge	I Tbsp.	65	8	2.0		
cream, Cool Whip, nondairy	I Tbsp.	12	1	1.0		
marshmallow fluff	I Tbsp.	60	15	0.0	♥	
pineapple	I Tbsp.	65	16	0.0	♥	

♥ = HEALTHY HEART FOOD   T = TRIGGER FOOD

Item	SERVING	CAL-ORIES	CARBS (g)	TOTAL FAT(g)	♥	T
strawberry	1 Tbsp.	60	15	0.0	♥	
Yogurt—regular, see our Dairy section						
Yogurt, frozen						
chocolate	½ cup	110	24	0.0	♥	T
peach	½ cup	100	23	0.0	♥	T
vanilla	½ cup	100	23	0.0	♥	T

VEGETABLES

Item	SERVING	CAL-ORIES	CARBS (g)	TOTAL FAT(g)	♥	T
Alfalfa sprouts	1 cup	10	1	0.0	♥	
Artichokes (1 large)	1 cup	55	12	0.0	♥	
Asparagus (6 spears)	1 cup	22	5	0.0	♥	
Bamboo shoots	1 cup	25	4	1.0		
Bean sprouts, mung	1 cup	30	6	0.0	♥	
Beets	1 cup	55	11	0.0	♥	T
Broccoli (1 spear)	1 cup	40	8	1.0		T
Brussels sprouts	1 cup	60	13	1.0	♥	T
Cabbage, Chinese, cooked						
cooked, Pak-choi	1 cup	20	3	0.0	♥	
fresh, Pe-tsai	1 cup	10	2	0.0	♥	
Cabbage, green						
cooked	1 cup	30	7	0.0	♥	
fresh	1 cup	15	4	0.0	♥	
Cabbage, red, fresh	1 cup	20	4	0.0	♥	
Cabbage, Savoy, fresh	1 cup	20	4	0.0	♥	
Carrots						
cooked (2 carrots)	1 cup	70	16	0.0	♥	T
fresh (2 carrots)	1 cup	30	7	0.0	♥	T
Carrot juice	1 cup	97	23	0.4	♥	T
Cauliflower	1 cup	30	6	0.0	♥	
Celery (1 stalk)	1 cup	5	1	0.0	♥	
Collards	1 cup	25	5	0.0	♥	
Corn						
canned, cream style	1 cup	185	46	1.0	♥	
canned, in water	1 cup	165	41	1.0	♥	T
fresh, cooked (2 ears)	1 cup	170	38	2.0	♥	T
frozen, cooked	1 cup	135	34	0.0	♥	T
Cucumber (1 medium)	1 cup	5	1	0.0	♥	
Dandelion greens	1 cup	35	7	1.0		

♥ = HEALTHY HEART FOOD   T = TRIGGER FOOD

Item	SERVING	CAL-ORIES	CARBS (g)	TOTAL FAT(g)	♥	T
Eggplant	1 cup	25	6	0.0	♥	T
Endive	1 cup	10	2	0.0	♥	
Artichoke, Jerusalem	1 cup	115	26	0.0	♥	
Kale	1 cup	40	7	1.0		
Kohlrabi, stems	1 cup	50	11	0.0	♥	
Lettuce						
butterhead, Boston (¼ head)	1 cup	5	1	0.0	♥	
cos (¼ head)	1 cup	10	2	0.0	♥	
iceberg (¼ head)	1 cup	20	3	1.0		
romaine (½ head)	1 cup	10	2	0.0	♥	
Mung bean, sprouted	1 cup	32	6	0.2	♥	
Mushrooms						
boiled/canned	1 cup	40	8	1.0		T
fresh	1 cup	20	3	0.0	♥	
sautéed in 2 Tbsp. oil	1 cup	320	12	28.2		T
Mustard greens	1 cup	20	3	0.0	♥	
Okra pods (3 pods)	1 cup	9	2	0.0	♥	
Onions						
cooked	1 cup	60	13	0.0	♥	T
fresh	1 cup	55	12	0.0	♥	T
Onion rings, breaded & cooked, frozen (5 rings)	1 cup	200	20	12.5		
Parsley (10 sprigs)	1 cup	5	1	0.0	♥	
Parsnips	1 cup	125	30	0.0	♥	
Pea pods, Chinese, cooked	1 cup	65	11	0.0	♥	T
Peas, green	1 cup	120	22	1.0	♥	
Peppers, hot chili (6 peppers)	1 cup	20	4	0.0	♥	
Peppers						
green						
raw	1 cup	20	4	0.0	♥	
sautéed w/2 Tbsp. oil	1 cup	270	6	27.2		
red						
raw	1 cup	20	4	0.0	♥	T
sautéed w/2 Tbsp. oil	1 cup	270	6	27.2		T
Plantain, cooked & sliced	1 cup	178	48	0.2	♥	
Potato salad	1 cup	360	28	21.0		
Potatoes						
au gratin						
from mix	1 cup	230	31	10.0		
homemade	1 cup	325	28	19.0		
baked w/skin (1 medium)	1 cup	220	51	0.0	♥	T
french fries						
oil fried (14 strips)	1 cup	224	28	11.2		

♥ = HEALTHY HEART FOOD   T = TRIGGER FOOD

Item	SERVING	CAL-ORIES	CARBS (g)	TOTAL FAT(g)	♥	T
oven-baked (14 strips)	1 cup	154	24	5.6		
hash browns	1 cup	340	44	18.0		
mashed w/milk	1 cup	160	37	1.0	♥	
mashed w/milk & margarine	1 cup	225	35	9.0		
scalloped	1 cup	210	26	9.0		
sweet potatoes						
candied (3 pieces)	1 cup	435	87	9.0	♥	
cooked, plain (1 medium)	1 cup	115	28	0.0	♥	T
Pumpkin, canned	1 cup	85	20	1.0	♥	T
Radishes, fresh (5 large)	1 cup	6	1	0.0	♥	
Sauerkraut	1 cup	45	10	0.0	♥	T
Seaweed, kelp, raw	1 oz.	10	3	0.0	♥	
Seaweed, Spirulina, dried	1 oz.	80	7	2.0		
Spinach						
cooked, frozen/canned	1 cup	45	8	0.0	♥	
creamed	1 cup	120	18	4.0		T
fresh	1 cup	10	2	0.0	♥	
Spinach souffle	1 cup	220	3	18.0		T
Squash, summer, cooked	1 cup	35	8	1.0		T
Squash, winter, cooked	1 cup	80	18	1.0	♥	T
Sweet potatoes						
candied (3 pieces)	1 cup	435	87	9.0	♥	
cooked, plain (1 medium)	1 cup	115	28	0.0	♥	T
Tomatoes						
canned	1 cup	50	10	1.0	♥	T
fresh (1 large)	1 cup	40	8	0.6	♥	T
Tomato juice						
canned	1 cup	40	10	0.0	♥	T
Hunt's, canned	1 cup	40	9	0.0	♥	T
Hunt's, canned, no salt added	1 cup	60	15	0.0	♥	T
Tomato paste	1 cup	220	49	2.0	♥	T
Tomato puree	1 cup	105	25	0.0	♥	T
Tomato sauce	1 cup	75	18	0.0	♥	T
Turnip greens	1 cup	30	6	0.0	♥	
Turnips, cooked	1 cup	30	8	0.0	♥	T
Vegetable juice, V-8	1 cup	47	11	0.0	♥	T
Vegetable juice cocktail	1 cup	45	11	0.0	♥	T
Vegetables, mixed, canned/frozen	1 cup	75	15	0.0	♥	T
Water chestnuts, canned	1 cup	70	17	0.0	♥	T

♥ = HEALTHY HEART FOOD   T = TRIGGER FOOD

Item	SERVING	CAL-ORIES	CARBS (g)	TOTAL FAT(g)	♥	T

Note: All foods listed in this section are vegetarian, nonmeat alternatives to animal products.

Item	SERVING	CAL-ORIES	CARBS (g)	TOTAL FAT(g)	♥	T
"Bacon," frozen						
Morningstar Farms	1 strip	27	1	2.0		T
Worthington Stripples	1 strip	40	2	2.3		T
Bacon bits, imitation						
Bac'N Pieces	1 tsp.	13	1	0.2	♥	
Bac* Os	1 tsp.	12	1	0.5		
Baked beans, canned						
plain	3 oz.	79	17	.4	♥	
w/miso, Health Valley	3 oz.	68	14	.8		
"Beef Pie," Worthington	3 oz.	135	30	6.0		
"Beef Steak"						
Worthington Prime Steakos	3 oz.	148	6	9.2		T
Worthington Stakelets	3 oz.	189	8	10.7		
"Beef Stew," Worthington	3 oz.	78	8	3.5		
"Beef," Worthington frozen						
roll	3 oz.	156	8	7.2		
Savory Slices	3 oz.	150	6	9.0		T
smoked	3 oz.	180	11	9.0		
"Bologna," Worthington Bologna	3 oz.	66	5	4.8		T
"Burger"						
frozen, Morningstar Farms	3 oz.	240	7	16.0		
mix (does not include fat for frying)						
Nature's Burger, barbeque	3 oz.	117	24	.8		T
Nature's Burger, original	3 oz.	152	21	4.0		T
Nature's Burger, pizza	3 oz.	121	24	1.0		T
w/tofu	3 oz.	125	12	4.8		
Burrito, chili	1	260	31	9.6		
Butter substitute						
sesame butter						
paste	1 Tbsp.	85	5	7.3		T
tahini, from toasted kernels	1 Tbsp.	89	3	8.1		T
tahini, from roasted kernels	1 Tbsp.	89	3	8.1		T
Cheese substitutes						
cheddar, from tofu	1 oz.	80	1	8.0		
cheddar, Sargento	1 oz.	90	1	6.0		
colby, Dorman's LoChol	1 oz.	90	1	6.0		
cream cheese, Tofutti	1 oz.	80	1	8.0		
mozarella, Sargento	1 oz.	80	1	6.0		

Item	SERVING	CAL-ORIES	CARBS (g)	TOTAL FAT(g)	♥	T
Muenster, Dorman's LoChol	1 oz.	100	1	7.0		
Swiss, Dorman's LoChol	1 oz.	100	1	7.0		
"Chicken"						
canned slices, Worthington	1 slice	45	1	4.0		
frozen, Worthington	3 oz.	280	17	19.0		T
frozen slices, Worthington	1 slice	65	2	4.5		
Morningstar Farms Country Crisp	1 patty	220	13	15.0		
Worthington FriChik	1 piece	90	2	6.5		
"Chicken Nuggets"						
homestyle, Morningstar Farms	3 oz.	250	18	16.0		
zesty, Morningstar Farms	3 oz.	280	17	19.0		
"Chicken Pie," Worthington	3 oz.	143	17	7.5		
"Chicken Roll," Worthington	3 oz.	189	5	12.0		T
"Chicken Sticks," Worthington	1 piece	110	4	7.0		
Chili						
spicy, Hain	3 oz.	64	12	0.4		
tempeh, spicy, Hain	3 oz.	64	9	1.6		
w/lentils, Health Valley	3 oz.	98	12	2.3		
Chow mein entree						
tofu & oil, Tofu Classic	½ cup	134	14	9.0		T
tofu, Tofu Classic	½ cup	110	14	6.0		T
"Corned Beef," Worthington	3 oz.	180	13	7.8		T
"Crab"	3 oz.	87	9	1.2	♥	T
Cream Substitute (nondairy)						
from frozen	1 tsp.	10	2	0.5		
liquid, Rich's Coffee Rich	1 tsp.	7	1	0.7		
powder						
Coffee-mate	1 tsp.	10	1	0.6		
Coffee-mate Lite	1 tsp.	8	2	0.5		T
Cremora	1 tsp.	10	1	0.6		
sour cream	1 Tbsp.	25	1	2.0		T
whipped topping						
frozen						
Cool Whip	1 Tbsp.	12	1	1.0		
Lite Cool Whip	1 Tbsp.	8	1	0.5		
most brands	1 Tbsp.	15	1	1.0		
pressurized	1 Tbsp.	10	1	1.0		
"Cutlet"						
regular, Worthington	3 oz.	92	4	1.9	♥	
multigrain, Worthington	3 oz.	83	6	0.9	♥	T

♥ = HEALTHY HEART FOOD T = TRIGGER FOOD

Item	SERVING	CAL-ORIES	CARBS (g)	TOTAL FAT(g)	♥	T
Egg substitute						
frozen						
Egg Beaters, Fleischmann's	¼ cup	25	1	0.0	♥	
Egg Watchers, tofutti	¼ cup	50	2	2.0		
Scramblers, Morningstar Farms	¼ cup	60	3	3.0		T
liquid	¼ cup	52	1	2.1		
mix, Tofu Scrambler w/butter	¼ cup	79	4	6.0		T
mix, Tofu Scrambler w/o butter	¼ cup	49	4	2.5		T
Egg roll, Worthington	1 roll	160	20	6.0		T
Enchilada entree	3 oz.	74	11	2.2		
"Frankfurter"						
Worthington Dixie Dogs	1 stick	200	21	10.0		
Worthington Leanies	1 link	100	2	6.0		T
Worthington Super-Links	1 link	100	3	7.0		
Worthington Veja-Links	1 link	70	2	5.0		
Hummus	½ cup	222	19	13.0		
Ice cream bars, substitute						
chocolate fudge, Good Humor	1	127	27	0.6	♥	
Cool Shark, Good Humor	1	68	17	0.1	♥	
Ice cream substitute						
all flavors, Lite Lite Tofutti	½ cup	90	20	0.4	♥	T
chocolate, Sealtest Free	½ cup	100	23	0.0	♥	T
vanilla, Sealtest Free	½ cup	100	24	0.0	♥	T
vanilla, Tofutti	½ cup	200	21	11.0		T
Lasagna entree, veg. w/tofu & sauce	½ cup	240	26	8.0		
Lentil dinner, canned w/vegs	3 oz.	64	7	1.6		
Lentil rice loaf, frozen	3 oz.	143	14	6.8		
Lentils, sprouted	½ cup	40	8	0.2	♥	
Little Caesar's meals sandwich	1	620	58	30.0		
"Lox," Mox Lox	3 oz.	50	6	1.6		T
Luncheon "meat"						
canned Worthington Numete	3 oz.	200	8	13.7		T
canned, Worthington Protose	3 oz.	200	10	8.9		T
Mayonnaise, substitute						
Hain Eggless	1 Tbsp.	110	0	12.0		
soybean	1 Tbsp.	35	2	2.9		

♥ = HEALTHY HEART FOOD   T = TRIGGER FOOD

Item	SERVING	CAL-ORIES	CARBS (g)	TOTAL FAT(g)	♥	T
sunflower	1 Tbsp.	71	1	8.0		
tofu	1 Tbsp.	40	1	4.0		
"Meatball," canned, Worthington	3 oz.	158	6	10.0		
Meat extender, soybean	3 oz.	264	33	2.4	♥	T
Milk substitute						
from soy milk	8 fl. oz.	79	4	4.6		
from vegetable oil	8 fl. oz.	136	16	16.0		T
Miso						
w/barley malt (mugi-koji)	3 oz.	168	24	3.6	♥	T
w/rice malt (kome-koji), dk. yellow	3 oz.	159	15	4.8		T
w/rice malt (kome-koji), sweet	3 oz.	186	30	2.4	♥	T
w/soybean malt (mame-koji)	3 oz.	186	9	11.7		T
Mung bean, sprouted	½ cup	16	3	0.1	♥	
Noodle						
Chinese cellophane	3 oz.	300	74	0.6	♥	
Chinese chow mein, dry	3 oz.	596	48	26.1		
Japanese soba, cooked	3 oz.	84	18	0.0	♥	
Japanese somen, cooked	3 oz.	87	18	0.0	♥	
Japanese Udon, cooked	2 oz.	87	18	0.5	♥	
Pizza, frozen, vegetable						
Celeste	¼ pie	310	28	16.0		
Celeste Pizza for One	1 pie	490	44	26.0		
Veg Deluxe, Stouffer's	½ pkg.	420	41	20.0		T
Plantain, cooked & sliced	½ cup	89	24	0.1	♥	
Potato pancake, homestyle	1	495	26	12.6		
"Salami"						
roll, Worthington	1 slice	45	2	2.5		
slices, Worthington	1 slice	40	2	2.0		
"Salmon, smoked," Mox Lox	3 oz.	50	6	1.6		T
"Sausage"						
links						
canned, Worthington	1	70	3	4.5		T
frozen, Morningstar Farms	1	63	1	4.7		
frozen, Worthington	1	63	1	4.7		
patties						
frozen, Morningstar Farms	1	95	2	6.0		
frozen, Worthington	1	105	2	7.0		
"Scallops"	3 oz.	84	9	0.3	♥	T

♥ = HEALTHY HEART FOOD   T = TRIGGER FOOD

Item	SERVING	CAL-ORIES	CARBS (g)	TOTAL FAT(g)	♥	T
Sesame butter						
paste	1 Tbsp.	85	5	7.3		T
tahini, from toasted kernel	1 Tbsp.	89	3	8.1		T
Sesame chips	½ cup	326	22	18.4		T
Sesame seeds, dried	½ cup	441	7	41.1		T
"Shrimp"	3 oz.	87	8	1.2	♥	T
Soybeans						
boiled from dry	½ cup	149	8	7.7		T
dry-roasted	½ cup	387	28	18.6		T
roasted	½ cup	405	29	21.8		T
Soy beverages						
carob, Ah Soy	8 fl. oz.	213	40	4.0	♥	
Soy Moo	8 fl. oz.	125	11	5.0		
vanilla, Ah Soy	8 fl. oz.	213	31	6.7		
Soy flour, raw	1 oz.	124	10	5.9		
Soy milk	8 oz.	79	4	4.6		
Soy sauce	1 Tbsp.	11	1	0.3		T
Tempeh	½ cup	165	14	6.4		T
Tempura batter, Golden Dipt	1 oz.	100	22	0.0	♥	
Teriyaki	1 Tbsp.	11	1	0.3		T
Tofu						
frozen, Natural Touch garden	1 patty	90	3	4.0		
frozen, Natural Touch Okara	1 patty	160	7	10.0		
raw, pasteurized (4 oz.)	1 patty	89	3	7.0		
Tofu spread, Natural Touch	1 Tbsp.	28	1	2.2		
"Tuna"	3 oz.	150	5	11.5		T
"Turkey"						
canned, Worthington	1 slice	65	2	4.5		
frozen, Worthington smoked	1 slice	45	1	3.0